Integrated Care Pathways

Senior commissioning editor: Mary Seager
Editorial assistant: Caroline Savage
Production controller: Anthony Read
Desk editor: Claire Hutchins
Cover designer: Fred Rose

Integrated Care Pathways: A Practical Approach to Implementation

Edited by

Sue Middleton and **Adrian Roberts**

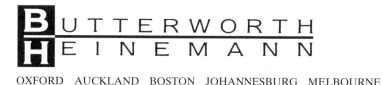

OXFORD AUCKLAND BOSTON JOHANNESBURG MELBOURNE NEW DELHI

Butterworth-Heinemann
Linacre House, Jordan Hill, Oxford OX2 8DP
225 Wildwood Avenue, Woburn, MA 01801–2041
A division of Reed Educational and Professional Publishing Ltd

℞ A member of the Reed Elsevier plc group

First published 2000

British Library Cataloguing in Publication Data
A catalogue record for this book is available from the British Library

Library of Congress Cataloguing in Publication Data
A catalogue record for this book is available from the Library of Congress

ISBN 0 7506 4087 1

Composition by Scribe Design, Gillingham, Kent, UK
Printed and bound in Great Britain by MPG Books Ltd, Bodmin, Cornwall

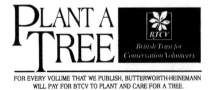

Contents

About the editors

Sue Middleton – Director, Integrated Care Associates
Sue is from a nursing and education background and has led a number of Welsh Office quality initiatives focusing on clinical effectiveness, clinical audit, care profiles and care pathways. She is a former integrated care facilitator within a Community and Mental Health Trust and an experienced trainer. She has delivered a number of clinical pathway training programmes on behalf of the Clinical Pathways Reference Centre, Wales and the King's Fund, London.

Adrian Roberts – Associate Director, Integrated Care Associates
Adrian is a qualified Projects in Controlled Environments (PRINCE) practitioner and is from an information management background.

Formerly a project manager with the NHS Benchmarking Reference Centre, he is also a qualified librarian. He has been actively involved in the development of quality improvement initiatives focusing on the application of care pathways, care packages, benchmarking and clinical process re-design.

Integrated Care Associates (ICA) was established in 1998 and provides facilitation, training and project management for health and social care organizations seeking to manage their service delivery by use of integrated care pathways. ICA also provide support services in research, diagnostic reviews and the development of good practice guidelines. The website address for ICA is www.integratedcareassociates.co.uk

Contributors

Leslie Braidwood
Dr Braidwood is a general practitioner based in Doncaster and APPROACH executive – Agreed Pathways and PROtocols for Accessing Care in Health.

Tracy P. Evans
Tracy is Integrated Pathway of Care Co-ordinator at Doncaster Royal Infirmary and Montagu Hospital NHS Trust.

Rhona Hotchkiss
Rhona is Director of the Nursing and Midwifery Practice Development Unit, Scottish Office.

Tom Jones
Tom is director of MJM Healthcare Solutions.

Denise Kitchiner
Dr Kitchiner is Consultant Paediatric Cardiologist at Royal Liverpool Children's Hospital NHS Trust.

Kathryn de Luc
Kathryn is an independent health care research consultant and committee member of the National Pathways Association.

Foreword

When I first started to use integrated care pathways (ICPs), there was little practical information available on their development and implementation. Most of the relevant literature originated in the United States and was not always applicable in an NHS setting. We set about developing ICPs – some worked and some failed, but we learnt from these experiences – experiences captured in this book. As ICPs have become increasingly popular and more Trusts are developing and using them, anyone starting out today has a much better chance of success from the start.

The introduction of clinical governance has led to increased interest in ICPs as the tool by which nationally defined guidelines and standards can be made locally applicable, leading to continuous quality improvement. Whilst research about the impact of ICPs is thin, there is increasing evidence from audit and evaluation in Trusts that ICPs lead to real improvements in standards and outcomes for patients.

This book is a practical guide to the development, implementation and evaluation of ICPs, written by people with understanding and experience. It provides an excellent basis for anyone wanting to know how to make ICPs work. It gives me pleasure to recommend it.

Dr Melanie Jayne Maxwell MBBS MRCPI MFPHM
Director of CPRU, Wirral Hospital NHS Trust

Acknowledgements

The editors would like to thank the following people and organizations for allowing us to share in their success.

- **Appendix 2: Integrated care pathway for 'cardiac' chest pain/suspected myocardial infarction**
  Alastair Miller, Consultant Physician/Clinical Director of Medicine, Sally Davis, clinical nurse specialist in coronary disease and Gill Price, ICP co-ordinator.
  Kidderminster Health Care NHS Trust.
- **Appendix 3: Integrated care pathway for day case cardiac catheters**
  Sue Jervis, Cardiac Directorate Manager and her team, Shirallee Jarret, ICP co-ordinator.
  Papworth Hospital NHS Trust.
- **Figure 7.3: Otitis media with effusion integrated pathway of care for children**
  The Doncaster Royal & Montagu Hospital.
- **Figure 6.10: Paediatric asthma pathway**
  Louisa Heaf and staff at Royal Liverpool Children's Hospital NHS Trust.
- **Figure 6.1: Sample medical assessment page** and **Figure 6.4: Sample multidisciplinary assessment page**
  Orthopaedic department and Julie Jones, Wrexham Maelor Hospital NHS Trust.
- **Figure 1.1: Sample pages from a pathway for suspected myocardial infarction**
  Glasgow Western Infirmary, clinical audit department.

Part One

WHAT ARE INTEGRATED CARE PATHWAYS?

1

Introduction

Sue Middleton and Adrian Roberts

Context

The NHS is undergoing a period of significant change. Patients are increasingly sophisticated consumers of health care and have correspondingly high expectations, placing greater demands on busy health professionals. A number of high-profile cases have helped to raise understandable concerns about the quality of care patients receive and its consistency from one part of the country to another. Differences in practice between clinicians and different organizations can lead to wide variations in both patient care and outcome. Patients are now also more likely to complain about poor treatment with claims for clinical negligence running at record levels.

Increasing pressure on the NHS, with more patients being treated than ever before, with an often-higher level of dependency, has also led to the development of considerable frustrations for clinical staff. Patients, for example, are often treated as 'outliers' on wards not suitable for their condition. Limitations in time and resources can also affect the ability of staff to deliver the standard of care they would like to see all their patients receive.

In this context, there is a new emphasis towards the provision of a controlled environment that delivers high quality, cost-effective care and minimizes potential risks and inappropriate costs (Ellis and Johnson, 1997). There are currently a number of NHS initiatives aimed at improving the quality of health care. These include the introduction of national service frameworks, the development of evidence-based health care and clinical effectiveness and a programme of continuous quality improvement through benchmarking. In addition, the emerging theme of clinical governance and the introduction of a national performance framework will increase the accountability of the NHS for its actions.

NHS organizations are also 'required' (NHS Wales, 1998) to examine new approaches to care which:

- focus on the patient's journey through the care process;
- are capable of creating alternatives to existing functional and organizational relationships;
- are open to testing and validation;
- are capable of developing process-based performance measures and clinical outcome measures; and
- integrate care across professional and organizational boundaries.

ICPs can be seen as one way of implementing these initiatives into everyday clinical practice. Throughout the UK it is estimated that more than 100 NHS trusts and other health care bodies use pathways as part of their clinical care. A National Pathways Association has been established to support users in England and Wales and has over 200 members. The Scottish Pathways Association has also been set up to support users in Scotland.

Integrated care pathways as a model of care

An ICP is an outline or plan of anticipated clinical practice for a group of patients (client group) with a particular diagnosis or set of symptoms. The ICP provides a multidisciplinary template of the plan of care, leading each patient towards a desired objective.

> An integrated care pathway determines locally agreed, multidisciplinary practice based on guidelines and evidence where available, for a specific patient/client group. It forms all or part of the clinical record, documents the care given and facilitates the evaluation of outcomes for continuous quality improvement.
>
> **National Pathways Association**

In simple terms, the ICP document is a matrix which places *interventions* (tasks) on one axis and time (hours, days, weeks) and milestones (specific stages of recovery) on the other.

The fundamental principle of ICPs is to make explicit the most appropriate care for a patient group, based on the available evidence and a consensus of best practice. The intention of ICPs is to ensure evidence-based care is delivered to the patient by the right individual, at the right time and in the right environment, helping to reduce unnecessary variations in treatment and outcome.

A number of elements make up the ICP model of care. These can be described as:

- patient groups
- scope
- multidisciplinary collaboration
- sequential and appropriate care
- patient-focused care
- single record of care
- analysis of variations.

Patient groups

Patient groups are groups of patients with similar clinical symptoms, requiring similar treatment, services and resources. ICPs are generally developed for high-volume and/or high-risk patient groups whose diagnosis, interventions, timelines and outcomes can be predicted (Currie and Harvey, 1997). Patient groups (see Table 1.1) can be organized around case types, specific disease categories, levels of dependence and by access routes into care (e.g. elective or emergency).

The success of an ICP is often dependent on the choice of client group together with the reasons why a particular group is chosen. Further guidance on choosing appropriate client groups can be found in **Chapter 5, Getting started**.

Scope

An ICP has a defined scope, including an agreed start and end point. The scope of the pathway provides a clear focus for it and helps to ensure the right patients are placed on the pathway. The scope of the ICP also influences which staff will be involved in its development and delivery and the desired objective of care for the chosen patient group.

Example: Paediatric asthma

Possible start point: Admission to A&E

Possible end point: Transfer to children's ward or discharge home

Further guidance on defining the scope of an ICP can be found in **Chapter 5, Getting started**.

Multidisciplinary collaboration

The use of ICPs requires multidisciplinary team working, bringing together all the professionals involved in delivering care to the chosen patient group. Each professional's role within the care cycle is clearly defined, helping to improve communication between professional groups and reducing areas of duplication. As patient outcomes are also specified in advance, each

Table 1.1 Sample patient groups

Monitoring
- *Pregnancy*
- *Insulin dependent diabetes*
- *Management of clinical depression in the community*
- *High blood pressure*
- *Terminal care*

Elective
- *Hip/knee replacement*
- *Cataract surgery*
- *Hysterectomy*
- *Repair of inguinal hernia*
- *Bronchoscopy*

Emergency
- *Stroke*
- *Myocardial infarction*
- *Acute asthma*
- *Acute appendicitis*
- *Aortic aneurysm*

member of the team (and the patient and their carers) have a clear idea of what is expected of them and for this reason, ICPs are often used as part of an orientation programme for new/bank staff or staff members on short rotation.

Example: Hip replacement

Primary health care team
GP, Practice nurse, Phlebotomist, Physiotherapist, Pharmacist, etc.

Social services
Social worker

Hospital team
Doctor(s), Nurse(s), Radiologist, Phlebotomist, Anaesthetist, Dietician, Therapist(s), Health care assistant(s), Pharmacist, etc.

Sequential and appropriate care

ICPs document the interventions necessary for the patient to progress along the pathway. They are recorded in sequence together with information on when the intervention is to take place, how it is to be achieved and by whom. The sequence of interventions is planned against a time-frame, often using days as a common unit of measurement as the patient moves from one stage of the pathway to the next. Initial development of ICPs has tended to focus on simple surgical procedures as a clearly logical sequence of events can be defined (Table 1.2).

For a more complex sequence of events, milestones or decision points can be used to represent the time-frame, as shown in Table 1.3.

The use of ICPs also demands that we examine the **appropriateness** of the care provided to the chosen patient group. Appropriateness is defined as 'suitable or proper' (Oxford English Dictionary) and can be determined by answering the following questions:

- What are the most appropriate interventions for the chosen patient group?
- When is the appropriate time to carry out these interventions?
- Where is the most appropriate place for these interventions to happen?
- Who is the best-qualified person to undertake these interventions?

Table 1.2 Typical surgical time-frame for hysterectomy

	Pre-op assessment	*Day of admission/ surgery*	*Post-op Day 1*	*Post-op Day 2*	*Post-op Day 3*	*Discharge Day 4*	*Out-patient appointment*
Assessment							
Investigation							
Medication							
Education							
Mobility							

Table 1.3 Typical time-frame for acute stroke

	Acute phase: assessment and investigation	*Monitoring phase*	*Rehabilitation phase in-patient*	*Rehabilitation phase out-patient (possible day hospital)*
Assessment				
Investigation				
Medication				
Education				
Mobility				

And:

- What evidence exists to support our answers to these four questions, in terms of robust research, national or local guidelines and protocols, etc?

Patient-focused

Traditional forms of service delivery have tended to be based around organizational structures. Services can often develop in an ad-hoc manner with no defined relationship between the different aspects of service delivery. Patients, for example, may need to see many different professionals, on different days, and in different departments.

ICPs place the patient at the centre of the care cycle. They encourage both professionals and organizations to view *'the patient's journey'* from a different perspective and to identify how the co-ordination of care and its consistency can be improved.

A number of ICPs are also being developed as education tools to provide patients with information on their condition and treatment. There is also an opportunity for patients to use ICPs as personal diaries, empowering them as active participants in their own care.

Single record of care

ICPs offer the opportunity to develop a single record of care. All staff involved in delivering care to the patient are required to record their input on the ICP document. The emphasis is on exception reporting against a pre-determined management plan, helping to reduce the length of time spent on documentation.

Full compliance with ICP documentation meets the requirements of the Clinical Negligence Scheme for Trusts and The Royal College of Nursing and Chartered Society of Physiotherapists standards for record keeping.

Analysis of variations

ICPs are not intended to compromise clinical judgement. Any member of the clinical team can deviate from the pathway if there is valid reason for doing so. The intention is for clinical freedom to be exercised according to the needs of the individual patient. Individual variations are actioned immediately and may mean the patient spends some time off the pathway, returning when the reason for the variation has been addressed or resolved.

Analysis of variations from the pathway through retrospective audit identifies trends in the delivery of care to the chosen patient group. The identification of trends helps to proactively manage clinical risk and allows the evaluation of care provided through the pathway. This information can be used to change the pathway as appropriate and complete the clinical audit cycle.

Benefits and limitations of ICPs

There are a number of specific benefits attributed to the use of ICPs. They can be described as follows:

- *Current practice is reviewed*: During the development of an ICP, the multidisciplinary team meet to establish current practice for the chosen patient group. Each professional describes his or her input into the care cycle. However, a baseline audit of a set of case notes for the patient group often shows that the perceptions of staff sometimes differ from reality. One reason for this may be the arrival of new junior doctors or bank staff who may not be familiar with the patient group or case type in question. The review of practice can also highlight problem areas and/or areas of duplication, allowing changes in practice to be made as appropriate.
- *Evidence is reviewed and incorporated, if appropriate*: ICPs offer a means of incorporating available evidence and national and local guidelines into everyday clinical care. Traditionally, guidelines are either kept on a shelf or pinned to a wall on the ward/back at base and may not be readily available to staff when they need them. Including this information in the ICP supports effective decision making. If there is no evidence available for the chosen patient group, the clinical team needs to reach a consensus of what constitutes *'best practice'*.
- *Variations in practice are justified*: The continuing emphasis on evidence-based health care is likely to mean that 'access to marginal options will inevitably reduce in future' (Belsey, 1997). However, the limited restric-

SUSPECTED MYOCARDIAL INFARCTION
OBJECTIVE:

Expected LOS: 6 days   **Actual LOS: days**

PATIENT DETAILS
Name:
Address:
Phone no:
DOB:
Hospital no:
Religion
Marital status:

ADMISSION DETAILS
Date:
Time:
Reason for admission:
Named nurse:
Consultant:
GP:
Admitted from:

ADMISSION OBSERVATIONS
BP:
Pulse:
Respiration:
Urinalysis:
BM:

PROVISIONAL DIAGNOSIS

DISCHARGE CRITERIA	**MET**	**DATE**
1.	❏	
2.	❏	
3.	❏	
4.	❏	

This pathway represents usual practice and variations are expected as clinicians use their own professional judgement.

Page 1 of

Figure 1.1 Sample pages from a pathway for suspected myocardial infarction. *Source*: Middleton, S. and Roberts, *A. Clinical Pathways Workbook*. Wrexham: VFM Unit, 1998

Patient
ID sticker   Day 2   WARD:

CLINICAL ASSESSMENT

MONITORING	*2 hrly*	*4 hrly*	*6 hrly*	*Comments*
Temp	❑	❑	❑	
Pulse	❑	❑	❑	
Resp.	❑	❑	❑	
B/P	❑	❑	❑	
ECG	❑	❑	❑	

INVESTIGATIONS

Repeat ECG   ❑

3rd cardiac enzyme   ❑   Results: _____

DIET: _____

DRUGS

1)

2)

3)

Analgesia required: yes ❑ no ❑   Adequate: yes ❑ no ❑

MANAGEMENT

Hygiene: shower if stable

Mobility: up to chair only

Dressing: remain in nightclothes

Lifestyle assessment: to be completed by nurse – refer to dietician: yes ❑ no ❑

Discharge plan: discuss follow up cardiac rehabilitation programme with patient

Nurse signature:

Figure 1.1 (*continued*) Sample pages from a pathway for suspected myocardial infarction. *Source*: Middleton, S. and Roberts, A. *Clinical Pathways Workbook*. Wrexham: VFM Unit, 1998

Patient ID sticker	Consultant: _____
	Age: _____
	Date of admission: / / Date of discharge: / /

VARIATIONS FROM PATHWAY

1. Patient condition	4. Medical omission/commission
2. Patient/family	5. Internal systems
3. Nurse omission/commission	6. External systems

Date	Time	Code	Variation	Sign	Action	Sign

© Western Glasgow Hospitals   Page 7 of

Figure 1.1 (*continued*) Sample pages from a pathway for suspected myocardial infarction. *Source*: Middleton, S. and Roberts, *A. Clinical Pathways Workbook*. Wrexham: VFM Unit, 1998

tions placed on clinical freedom by ICPs are created from the clinical evidence base. Variations from the pathway are justified by the needs of the individual patient and not through personal preference or custom.

By defining what is expected to happen to a particular patient group, clinical problems can be identified earlier, allowing quicker decisions to be made on the alternative course(s) of action.

- *Multidisciplinary communication is improved*: ICPs aim to improve practice 'through communication among clinicians in one discipline, between disciplines and between staff groups and patients' (Hotchkiss, 1997). Documenting practice in the ICP document co-ordinates the approach between the different professions and agencies involved in delivering care.
- *Client satisfaction is improved*: Several studies have suggested that patient satisfaction is improved by using ICPs (e.g. Stead et al., 1995). Patients on ICPs feel better informed about their care, are encouraged to ask questions about it and are more likely to be satisfied with the responses they receive from medical and nursing staff. Some sites are actively developing 'patient pathways' to assist in this process.

Patients are also provided with realistic expectations as to their condition and their expected progress. Discharge planning is begun on the day of admission/or with first contact with community services and patients and their carers are given a clear idea of the milestones they will need to reach before discharge.

- *Clinical outcomes are improved*: An increasing number of studies are also suggesting that clinical outcomes are improved by using ICPs (Hoffman, 1997; Ogilvie-Harris et al., 1993; Weilitz and Potter, 1993). These outcomes are also defined in advance, and agreed with the patient and carer. Milestones are used to measure the patient's progress along the pathway and this information can also be used to measure actual against expected progress.
- *Documentation is reduced*: It is estimated that clinicians spend up to 25 per cent of their time collecting and using information and 15 per cent of hospital resources are spent in gathering information (Audit Commission, 1995). Studies have shown that ICPs reduce the time spent on documentation (Turbo, 1993) and compliance with ICPs meets professional standards for record keeping.

- *Clinical staff*: ICPs help ensure that the care that clinical staff would like their patients to receive is delivered. An accurate record of clinical care is produced, with all variations from the expected clearly recorded. The use of ICPs for common conditions also allows more time to be devoted to the more complex patient.
- *Clinical pathways can be used to demonstrate the quality and appropriateness of care*: ICPs spell out the agreed standards that both the health care provider and clinicians seek to achieve, standards against which the actual care delivered can be measured. In terms of the need for providers to assess their common clinical procedures, the baseline reviews required for the development of pathways can help to provide a new focus for improvements in patient care. Analysis of variations provides concurrent and retrospective information for clinical audit, quantifying patient outcomes and explaining lengths of stay for different case types, changes in practice and the introduction of new guidelines. Evidence also suggests that ICPs can minimize duplications in care and reduce length of stay, thereby decreasing costs and improving patient flow.

The use of ICPs may also lead to 'evidence based commissioning' allowing more appropriate targeting of staff and other resources.

Critical success factors

For the benefits of ICPs to be realized, a number of critical success factors need to be addressed. These are the characteristics or variables that have a direct influence on the successful development and implementation of ICPs.

The identified success factors are:

- Commitment is demonstrated at senior management and clinical levels.
- ICPs are included as part of an organizational quality programme.
- Pathways are 'owned' by clinical staff and are completed by all the staff involved.

- Pathways are based on available evidence and best practice and include milestones and expected outcomes.
- Variations are collated and analysed and fed back to clinical staff.
- There is a rolling programme of education and support.

Limitations

There are two main limitations currently associated with the use of ICPs. These are:

- *Complex clients*: To date, major developments in ICPs have focused on the treatment of more predictable surgical procedures and some common medical conditions. However, some organizations have actively begun to develop ICPs for more complex, unpredictable patients, e.g. elderly frail clients in the community and patients with severe mental illness, and to extend pathways across acute and community care. The challenge exists to establish whether ICPs can successfully be used to manage these patients.
- *Evaluation*: A need exists for a formal scientific evaluation to be undertaken to establish the full impact of using ICPs in the UK. Current evidence relating to the success of ICPs is based on (1) local studies, (2) satisfaction surveys and (3) anecdotal evidence.

Conclusion

ICPs are important because they offer a vehicle to address a number of important issues currently facing the NHS. These include:

- the emergence of clinical governance and the development of new national performance frameworks;
- the need to incorporate evidence into practice;
- the use of outcome measures and clinical benchmarking to achieve measurable improvements in care;
- the development of multi-agency working and the use of 'care partnerships';
- active patient involvement in their own care;
- the development of appropriate risk management strategies to reduce litigation and claims of clinical negligence.

References

Audit Commission (1995) *For your information: a study of information management and systems in the acute hospital*. London, HMSO.

Belsey, Johnathan (1997) Should we fear managed care. *Journal of Managed Care*, 1(1), 12–14.

Currie, L. and Harvey, G. (1997) *The origins and use of care pathways in the USA, Australia and the United Kingdom*. Oxford, RCN Institute, Report no 15.

Ellis, B.W. and Johnson, S. (1997) A clinical view of pathways of care in disease management. *International Journal of Health Care Quality Assurance*, 10(2), 61–6.

Hoffman, P. (1997) Critical Path Method: An important tool for co-ordinating clinical care. *Journal of Quality Improvement*, 19(7), 235–46.

Hotchkiss, R. (1997) Managing care: integrated care pathways. *Research*, 2(1).

NHS Wales (1998) *Putting patients first*. Cardiff, Welsh Office.

Ogilvie-Harris, D., Botsford, D. and Worden Hawkes, R. (1993) Elderly patients with hip fractures: improved outcome with the use of care maps with high-quality medical and nursing protocols. *Journal of Orthopaedic Trauma*, 17(5), 428–37.

Trubo, R. (1993) If this is cookbook medicine, you may like it. *Medical Economics*, 69, 69–82.

Stead, L., Arthur, C. and Cleary, A. (1995) Do multi-disciplinary pathways of care affect patient satisfaction? *Health Care Risk Report*, November, 13–15.

Weilitz, P. and Potter, P. (1993) A managed care system: financial and clinical evaluation. *Journal of Nursing Administration*, 23(11), November.

Part Two

WHY INTRODUCE INTEGRATED CARE PATHWAYS?

2

ICPs and quality: the use of ICPs to facilitate a clinically effective service

Sue Middleton and Adrian Roberts

Introduction

The NHS has seen, in recent years, an increasing emphasis placed on quality management and the 'delivery' of quality health care. Quality management has been presented as the means of ensuring the NHS is able to rise to new challenges created by advances in technology and an expanding client base with increasingly sophisticated expectations of public services. Successive governments, keen to transfer the benefits realized from industry and the service sector to the NHS, have promoted a number of different quality initiatives, ranging from 'The Patient's Charter' to self-assessment, benchmarking and clinical effectiveness.

The term 'quality' remains difficult to define in the context of the management and delivery of health services as it is complicated by the following observations:

- Quality is not an absolute concept and it is therefore subjective rather than objective, e.g. different people may have different perceptions as to what constitutes quality – clinicians, managers, commissioners, politicians, patients and their carers.
- People's perceptions of quality may be dependent on their prior expectations and experiences.

Quality is perhaps most commonly defined as 'a degree or standard of excellence' (Collins English Dictionary), and it is certainly easier to understand when there is a standard to relate it to. In essence, quality can actually be seen to consist of a number of components that seek to ensure that the right people receive the right services, at the right time, to the right standard(s).

Key components of quality

- Establishing a baseline, analysing strengths and weaknesses, establishing desired outcomes – setting standards.
- Developing an action plan, implementing changes, service delivery – delivering high quality services.
- Reviewing actual performance against desired outcomes – performance monitoring.

The number of different quality management techniques on offer has meant that quality activity within NHS organizations has tended to be disparate, with one initiative often replaced by another before it has been completed. It can be argued, however, that the focus of quality initiatives has changed from an over-emphasis on organizational structure to concentrate on 'people' and the process and outcome of clinical/non-clinical care.

In terms of the level of service we seek to provide, it is clear that quality management has an important role to play in ensuring that all patients receive the high quality care they are 'entitled' to. What is less clear is how the lessons and results of the wide range of quality activity can be consistently applied in everyday practice. *This chapter explores the role ICPs can play in supporting the quality agenda, particularly within the context of the emerging theme of 'clinical governance'.*

Range of quality management techniques – examples

Quality frameworks
- Accreditation schemes, e.g. HQS, Health Services Accreditation, Hospital Accreditation Framework, Charter Mark, etc.
- Total quality management
- European Foundation for Quality Management (EFQM) framework
- ISO 9000
- Continuous quality improvement (CQI)

People
- Investors in People (IIP)

Process and outcome of health care
- Audit
- Benchmarking
- Clinical process re-design
- Re-engineering

The quality agenda

Recent consultation documents in England, Scotland, Wales and Northern Ireland (Department of Health, 1998b) have established a new quality agenda for the NHS, emphasizing the 'quality' of care delivered by participating organizations and their employees in preference to 'the counting of numbers, of measuring activity, of logging what could be logged' (Department of Health, 1998a). This agenda brings together a number of both new and existing quality initiatives into a framework for improvement, based on the three main components of quality:

- setting standards
- delivery of high quality services
- effective monitoring of performance.

Setting quality standards

The intention of the new quality agenda is to set a series of national standards for NHS services, supported by appropriate evidence-based guidance. The development of these standards will be facilitated by the National Institute for Clinical Excellence (NICE) and a set of National Service Frameworks outlining what services patients can expect to receive (and to what standards) from the NHS in major care areas/disease groups. The first four National Service Frameworks focus on coronary heart disease, mental health, children's intensive care and cancer services.

Delivery of high quality services

The delivery of high quality services at local level will be driven by the process of clinical governance (together with a statutory duty of quality) and supported by the twin themes of 'life-long learning' and 'professional self-regulation'.

Effective monitoring of performance

Compliance with national standards and the delivery of services will be monitored in three ways: (1) the Commission for Health Improvement will provide independent assessment of local action and visit all NHS trusts in a rolling review programme; (2) the national performance framework will assess how well each part of the NHS is delivering quality services against six key areas; and (3) the annual national patient survey will provide feedback on all aspects of NHS care 'from food to pain relief'.

Clinical governance

Clinical governance is the driving force behind the new quality agenda. It is intended to operate predominantly at local service level combining local responsibility with national quality standards. It is defined as:

> a framework through which NHS organisations are accountable for continuously improving the quality of their services and safeguarding high standards of care by creating an environment which excellence in clinical care will function. (NHS Wales, 1999a)

In essence, clinical governance can be seen as a quality framework (with similarities, for example, to the European Foundation for Quality Management *EFQM* framework) which can be used to co-ordinate disparate quality initiatives and the process of change. This allows organizations to use a number of different quality 'tools' appropriate to the service area under investigation or the nature of the problem(s) to be tackled.

Clinical governance

The clinical governance framework will:
- build on the best traditions of professional self-regulation and the principles of performance review
- strengthen existing systems for quality control, based on clinical standards, evidence-based practice and learning the lessons of poor performance.

Key components of the framework will include:
- a comprehensive programme of quality improvement activity (such as clinical audit and evidence-based practice) and processes for monitoring clinical care using effective information and clinical record systems
- clear policies aimed at managing risk, including procedures that support professional staff in identifying and tackling poor performance
- clear lines of responsibility and accountability for the overall quality of clinical care.

The development and use of ICPs can be seen as one such 'tool' to support the implementation of clinical governance. The main components of clinical governance are:

1. A comprehensive programme of quality improvement activities.
2. Clear policies aimed at managing risk.
3. Clear lines of responsibility and accountability for the overall quality of clinical care.

A comprehensive programme of quality improvement activities

A comprehensive programme of quality improvement activities should include:

- Full participation by all clinical staff in audit programmes;
- evidence-based practice supported and applied routinely in every-day practice;
- ensuring the clinical standards of National Service Frameworks and NICE recommendations are implemented;
- workforce planning and development (i.e. recruitment and retention of appropriately trained workforce), fully integrated within the NHS organization's service planning;

- effective monitoring of clinical care with high quality systems for clinical record keeping and the collection of relevant information;
- processes for assuring the quality of clinical care are in place and integrated with the quality programme for the organization as a whole.

Full participation by all clinical staff in audit programmes

Audit is an integral feature of the clinical effectiveness cycle and can be defined as: 'the systematic critical analysis of the quality of care, involving the procedures and processes used for diagnosis, intervention and treatment, the use of resources and the resulting outcome and quality of life as assessed by both professionals and patients' (Department of Health, 1989).

The key to successful audit is the 'audit cycle' which consists of the following stages:

1. negotiating standards
2. observing practice
3. measuring performance
4. implementing possible changes
5. reviewing and repeating stages 1–5.

Concerns relating to the effectiveness of audit exercises relate to the time required by clinicians to participate, difficulties in collecting the relevant data and how often the 'audit cycle' is successfully completed resulting in actual changes in clinical practice.

ICPs can act as a framework for clinical audit, providing both 'real-time' and retrospective data for audit purposes. The monitoring of actual interventions and their relationship with patient outcomes, together with the analysis of variations from the expected, are key elements of the ICP approach and this information can be used to inform 'every-day' practice. In terms of audit, the ICP acts as the 'standard' or 'standards' against which actual practice is judged. The identification of trends which deviate from this 'standard' allow changes and revisions to be made to the pathway as appropriate, ensuring that clinical practice is amended as required and helping to complete the audit cycle.

Evidence-based practice supported and applied routinely in every-day practice

A key component of the development of clinically effective practice is the use of evidence.

The intention of evidence-based practice is to ensure that:

- treatments that have little or no benefit, or are shown by evidence to be harmful are stopped
- treatments that are proved to be effective are provided to all that need them, and
- when decisions have to be made on priorities, evidence of effectiveness plays an important part in the decision-making process (NHS Wales, 1998).

As with clinical audit, evidence-based practice is based on a cycle made up of the following stages:

1. evidence-based information is used
2. to inform evidence-based practice
3. which is monitored and evaluated and (go to step 1).

There are a number of problems associated with the use of evidence-based practice. There appears to be a general lack of confidence about obtaining and handling evidence and concerns also exist as to whether the use of such evidence is appropriate in all local clinical settings. It is certainly true that the development of National Service Frameworks and the role of NICE in 'testing what works' will improve access to the available evidence but a vehicle is still required to implement evidence into routine practice and to ensure its use is effective at the level of individual clinical teams.

The baseline review of current practice required to develop an ICP enables the clinical team to ask questions about the appropriateness of particular investigations or treatments and to test the clinical process against the evidence base. Effective practice as proved by robust evidence can be incorporated into the pathway documentation ensuring its use by the clinical team on a day-to-day basis. The routine monitoring of patient outcomes and analysis of variations from the expected encouraged by ICPs also allows the clinical team to make a judgement as to whether the use of this evidence is appropriate to their local clinical setting.

In addition, there are many clinical situations for which robust evidence does not exist and an alternative must be considered. In these situations, ICPs encourage the clinical team to reach a consensus on what constitutes best practice for the chosen patient group and to identify how this differs from existing patterns of care. The ICP developmental process can also act as a sound basis for a benchmarking exercise to compare forms of service delivery and treatment patterns between different clinicians within the same organization and with other organizations.

Ensuring the clinical standards of National Service Frameworks and NICE recommendations are implemented
Whilst local ownership of the practice encapsulated in the pathway is a critical factor in their successful use, ICPs are certainly a convenient framework for ensuring the integration of recommended service patterns and nationally defined standards. The use of standards is a routine feature of ICPs, both as milestones to measure the progress of the patient from day-to-day and in terms of the

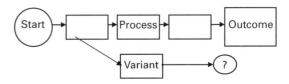

Figure 2.1 Recognized variation in the clinical process – same outcome?

outcomes the patient is 'expected' to achieve. The definition of standards and outcomes within ICPs can be informed with reference both to National Service Frameworks and NICE, together with information derived from clinical audit, accreditation and other quality initiatives.

Workforce planning and development (i.e. recruitment and retention of appropriately trained workforce) fully integrated within the NHS organization's service planning
The development of ICPs defines the roles and responsibilities of each member of the clinical team involved in providing care to the chosen patient group. This can help to identify both the numbers and skill-mix of staff required for the optimum delivery of care and any training required by staff (particularly junior doctors, staff on short rotation and bank staff) to fulfil their responsibilities.

Table 2.1 UKCC standards for record keeping and pathway compliance

UKCC standard	ICP	Comments
Concise	✔	ICP documentation outcome based and uses exception reporting
Comprehensive	✔	Covers the complete patient episode
Sequential	✔	Management and interventions recorded sequentially
Signed	✔	All interventions signed by responsible staff
Unambiguous	✔	Outcome based/exception reporting
Up-to-date	✔	ICPs completed in 'real time'
Evaluated	✔	Routine analysis of variations

Effective monitoring of clinical care with high quality systems for clinical record keeping and the collection of relevant information

In terms of high quality systems for record keeping, ICPs offer the opportunity to introduce a single, comprehensive record of care that accurately reflects the complete patient episode. In simple terms, the ICP ensures that the treatment the patient receives is reported, together with any deviations from the expected care plan and the reasons for these deviations. The ICP approach is also based on the information it is relevant to collect rather than what is easy to collect. Full compliance by all staff with the pathway ensures that ICPs meet the UKCC standards for record keeping (Table 2.1).

Processes for assuring the quality of clinical care are in place and integrated with the quality programme for the organization as a whole

ICPs have the potential to act as the integrated system for assuring the quality of clinical care. Their use encourages the routine assessment of patient outcomes together with any identified standards and milestones as defined within the pathway and in this way provides a link between the 'inputs' (the process of care) and the 'outputs' (the results of care) of all clinical activity managed through ICPs. This allows a judgement to be made on the impact of clinical care and its *clinical effectiveness*, which in basic terms can be described as the difference between what would have occurred naturally and what happens as a result of the care the patient receives.

ICPs also help to demonstrate the quality and appropriateness of care based on activities specifically related to the patient. In terms of assuring the overall quality of care, with a particular focus on common clinical procedures, the baseline reviews required for the development of ICPs helps to identify strengths and weakness within the system and a focus for improvement efforts. Routine analysis of variations from the expected and monitoring of the patient outcomes agreed in the ICP also helps to ensure that this assessment remains a dynamic process with changes in practice introduced as and when they are required.

Clear policies aimed at managing risk

In keeping with other quality initiatives, clinical risk management can be seen as a 'cycle' consisting of the following activities:

1. Baseline self-assessment undertaken to identify risks.
2. Programmes in place to manage identified risks.
3. Critical incident reporting of all adverse events.
4. Act on step 3 (return to step 1).

The evaluation of current practice undertaken during the 'getting started' phase of developing an ICP can be used to identify areas of risk and to ensure that appropriate management strategies are included in the pathway documentation. Variations from the expected plan of care help to identify potential adverse events in 'real time', allowing the clinical team to take the appropriate course of action to minimize their eventuality. Retrospective analysis of these variations will also highlight new areas of risk as they emerge, enabling the clinical team to make amendments to the plan of care as they are needed.

Legal issues

In cases of clinical negligence, the *defendant* (e.g. Health Authority, NHS Trust) is liable if they are at fault. They are deemed to be at fault if through acts or omissions they cause damage that is reasonably foreseeable. In addition, there are three cardinal principles in the law of negligence and all must be present before negligence can be established:

- There must be a duty of care imposed on the defender.
- There must be a failure on the part of the defender to comply with that duty of care.
- The damage or injury must have arisen out of the breech in the duty of care.

A duty of care exists where an injury to one party is a reasonably foreseeable consequence of the actions of another. The existence of a duty of care between a doctor and patient is therefore not usually questioned.

The standard of care that is applied in negligence cases is the standard of the '*reasonable man*'. The characteristics of a 'reasonable man' are generally established by assessing:

- knowledge at the time
- activity being performed
- importance of the objective to be achieved.

To determine the standard of care various factors have to be weighed in balance. The court examines existing practices to determine whether they are safe, the seriousness of the consequences, the difficulty of putting it right and the expense involved.

The test to be applied in all cases of medical negligence was established in 1955:

> In the realm of diagnosis and treatment there is ample scope for genuine difference of opinion and one man is clearly not negligent merely because his conclusion differs from that of other professional men, nor because he has displayed less skill or knowledge than others would have shown. The true test for establishing negligence in diagnosis or treatment on the part of a doctor is whether he has been proved to be guilty of such failure as no doctor of ordinary skill would be guilty if acting with ordinary care (Lord President Clyde: Hunter v. Hanley 1955 SC).

The test involves asking three questions:

- Was there a normal practice?
- Was it followed?
- If not, was the course adopted one which no professional of ordinary skill acting with ordinary care would have taken?

In these terms, it is clear that credible defence expert evidence should be sufficient to defend a claim of medical negligence, irrespective of the weight of evidence presented by the claimant.

In clinical negligence cases the relevant medical records will need to be scrutinized and the appropriate medical, nursing and therapy personnel identified. Reports must be obtained from these staff and also from the consultant in charge.

ICPs can be seen as an important tool in cases of clinical negligence as they provide evidence of co-ordinated approach to health care by:

- spelling out the agreed standards that both the health care provider and clinicians look to achieve, standards against which the actual care delivered can be measured (*normal practice*);
- providing an accurate and comprehensive record of the complete episode of care (*was this practice followed?*);
- detailing all variations from the expected care plan, including the course of action taken and the reason(s) why the alternative was chosen (*was the course of action undertaken one which no professional of ordinary skill acting with ordinary care would have taken?*)

Concerns have been expressed that non-compliance to ICPs could be used against the hospital/clinicians in malpractice claims but given the individual discretion that must be allowed in each pathway's application to specific patients, this seems unlikely.

Clear lines of responsibility and accountability for the overall quality of clinical care

Clinical governance intends to improve the accountability for the overall quality of clinical care by:

- making the NHS Trust Chief Executive ultimately responsible for assuring the quality of services provided by the trust;
- ensuring a designated senior clinician is responsible for ensuring that systems for clinical governance are in place and monitoring their continued effectiveness;

- requiring that formal arrangements for NHS/Local Health Group boards to discharge their responsibilities on clinical quality are in place;
- ensuring that regular reports to NHS boards on the quality of clinical care are given the same importance as the monthly financial report and that an annual report on clinical governance is produced.

Whilst these arrangements may clarify the overall lines of accountability for the quality of clinical care, it can be argued that accountability can only be improved at this level by reinforcing individual responsibility at the level of clinical teams. The nature of ICPs supports this process; individual roles and responsibilities are clearly defined with each member of the clinical team aware of both their own and their colleagues' input into the care cycle. Each member of the clinical team is given a clear idea of what is expected of them in order for the patient to achieve the desired outcome(s) specified in the ICP.

Conclusions

This chapter has shown how ICPs can help meet many of the requirements of clinical governance. By placing ICPs at the heart of quality initiatives, organizations are given the means to:

- identify the strengths and weaknesses within areas of clinical activity and service delivery and the scope for improvement (the baseline assessment);
- ensure that a planned quality improvement or change in clinical practice is implemented and *results* in the desired change (monitoring progress);
- make comparisons between clinical teams within the same organization and between a

local service and its counterparts elsewhere to identify scope for improvement (benchmarking and process redesign);
- provide information to the public about the quality of services provided (openness and public accountability);
- monitor variations from the expected and adverse outcomes of care (early warning of changes required in practice and serious failures) (adapted from NHS Wales, 1999b).

ICPs have close links with the quality cycle, if it is described in terms of *what do we do, how do we do it, can we do it better and how do we do it better* (Wilson, 1997). In addition, ICPs have natural links with a wide range of quality initiatives, including:

- clinical effectiveness and evidence-based practice
- clinical audit
- benchmarking; and
- process re-design.

References

Department of Health (1989) *Working for patients. Medical Audit – Working Paper 6. The Health Service, Caring for the 1990s.* London, HMSO.

Department of Health (1998a) *A first class service: quality in the NHS.* London, HMSO, p.1.

Department of Health (1998b) *The new NHS, modern, dependable.* London, HMSO.

NHS Wales (1998) *Nursing, Midwifery and Health Visiting Advisers for Clinical Effectiveness: Resource Directory.* November, p.15.

NHS Wales (1999a) *Clinical Governance: Quality Care and Clinical Excellence.* Cardiff, Welsh Office.

NHS Wales (1999b) *Putting Patients First. Clinical Governance. Quality Care and Clinical Excellence – Executive Summary.* Cardiff, Welsh Office, p.7.

Wilson, J. (1997) Introduction to integrated care management – introducing multidisciplinary pathways of care into an organization through project, risk and change management. In Wilson, J. (ed.), *Integrated Care Management: The Path to Success.* Oxford, Butterworth–Heinneman, p.21.

3

Effectiveness: the use of ICPs to facilitate a cost-effective service

Tom Jones

Introduction

Whilst the introduction of the new quality agenda has produced a shift in emphasis away from monitoring financial information and league tables towards the delivery of quality health care, the reality remains that the NHS is working with limited resources. Budgets for both the public and independent health sector may continue to grow, but demand still exceeds capacity and a 'bottomless pit' of finance does not exist. Within these constraints it is clear that 'efficiency' and 'cost-effectiveness' remain an integral feature of the quality equation. Indeed, the use of evidence-based practice often takes account of the clinical effectiveness of different treatments and interventions related to their costs.

The search for an increasingly cost-effective health service will continue and within this context the ICP approach offers a framework for cost-effectiveness based on:

- linking best patient outcomes with the resources needed to change them;
- incorporating best practice consistently;
- ensuring that patients are treated without unnecessary delays;
- connecting health care professionals and other resources efficiently;
- minimizing waste and improving resource allocation;
- optimizing costs along the whole health care continuum;
- matching costs to sustainable, demanding standards;
- deriving costs from information relevant to clinicians;
- controlling costs to sustain best standards;
- requiring active care management to sustain cost-effective standards, and

- offering benefits in improved financial performance.

Properly costed ICPs also offer choices about the optimum configuration of resources to meet patient needs. For example, given information on (1) relative benefits derived from evidence, (2) proper linkages between related services and (3) options for costs, decisions within an ICP for the most appropriate setting for out-patient clinics (or rehabilitation services, continuing care, etc.) can transcend boundaries between:

- primary health care teams (PCHT)
- community hospitals/services
- independent services
- voluntary services, and
- district general hospitals.

In keeping with the concept of quality, the question of cost-effectiveness can be seen from a number of perspectives, which in terms of the health service primarily equates to:

- patients
- providers, and
- commissioners.

This chapter explores the potential for using ICPs to facilitate a cost-effective health service from each of these different perspectives.

Patients

Patients see and experience health care as a range of health care professionals, services and facilities designed to combine to meet their individual needs. The effective integration of these components is identified by the ICP. Unfortunately, this does not always match the way that NHS services are currently

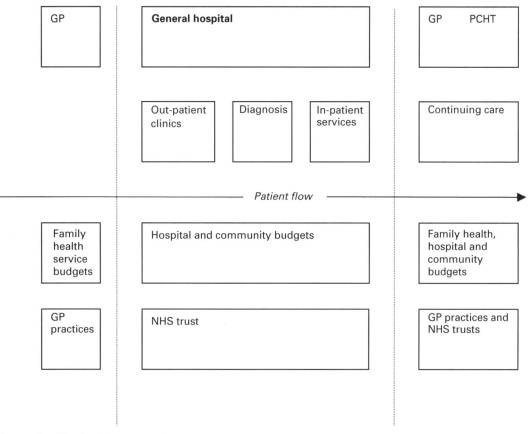

Figure 3.1 The health care continuum

organized or financed, creating an immediate potential culture clash that has to be resolved to improve cost-effective health care. A simple model of the current most common health care continuum (Figure 3.1) shows that patient flow cuts through the NHS organizational and financial structure *and* does not follow it.

As patients 'take up' health care, the professionals they come into contact with often work in different settings and organizations. Each setting or organization will have its own financial and budget regime and this can render the transfer of resources to match improvements in patient care quite challenging.

Any attempt to improve the cost-effectiveness of health care must deal with these institutional boundaries. As ICPs identify the scope to transfer effective patient care to more cost-effective settings, the real

resources and money to support them must transfer too. In a largely cash-limited NHS, this means a transfer from one part of the health continuum to another, and often one organization to another.

The patient perspective confirms the need to stretch the costing structure and methodology of ICPs across the full health care continuum. One way to achieve this is to incorporate only the direct costs associated with an ICP. Some of this can be released and aligned with the ICP, with separate components of care offered in the most effective setting. This requires a separate analysis of the indirect institutional costs, especially those associated with the fixed assets costs of health care. These cannot be released or moved, either on the same timescale or in the same way as the direct costs, and creates a challenge for providers to respond creatively.

Providers

NHS trusts and GP practices are the main NHS providers although the independent and voluntary sectors also provide health care and social services can provide care that contributes to cost-effectiveness. Using ICPs to improve cost-effectiveness could lead each service provider to:

- transfer resources and money within their directorates or departments;
- reduce the workload and costs of their activities;
- improve their resource utilization;
- reduce the costs of their performance;
- transfer resources and money to another organization in the NHS;
- transfer resources and money to another organization outside the NHS;
- make cost-effective use of extra resources and money received.

The concept and design of ICPs is entirely consistent with a standard costing methodology and its variance analysis. This has previously been established by a joint study undertaken by the Association of Chartered Certified Accountants and the National Pathways Association (ACCA and NPA, 1999). This study set out the components of an ICP model as a blend of several techniques pursued around the patient (Figure 3.2).

The techniques in this model are applied and developed to deal with separate dimensions of patient care. When they can be combined into a single setting, they offer the potential to be comprehensively patient focused and cost-effective.

Many of these techniques are emerging in the NHS and need to be developed as part of an improved patient focus. However, some of the techniques seem to be taking very different perspectives. It is only when they can be managed as a whole that a complete patient view can be achieved. In particular, enabling health care professionals to achieve quality goals and improve resource utilization requires information and knowledge for decision taking. The aim is to improve the relationships between the factors in the model. A cost model for providers proposed by the ACCA and NPA is shown in Figure 3.3.

In managing health care for improved cost-effectiveness, clinicians, managers and commissioners will need integrated information. The structure of ICPs is entirely consistent with standard costing techniques. They

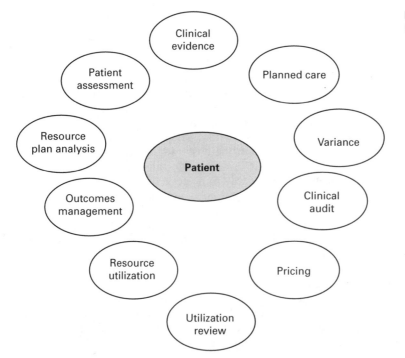

Figure 3.2 Patient-focused ICP model

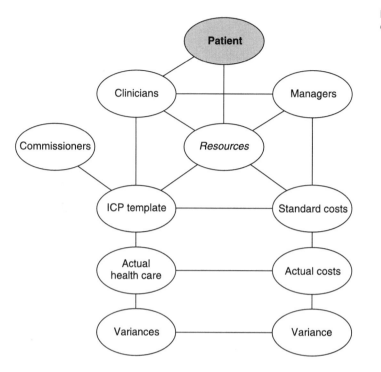

Figure 3.3 A cost model for health care providers

are both derived from agreed standards and both can have actual costs that differ from these standards. They both also provide information that allows these variances to be analysed. Using them together supports decisions about the standard of care to be provided at various levels of cost. These decisions can also be expressed in terms that are directly relevant to patient care and ensure that managing the resources for health care can match the management of its costs.

Options to change the roles of some health care professionals, such as by multi-skilling, can also be determined in this setting. The impact of changes on the cost base can be assessed against the scope to reduce, release and redeploy resources to other parts of the ICP. Focusing on the patient and supporting health care professionals and managers with consistent information about quality and costs enhances the scope to improve cost-effectiveness.

An extremely beneficial feature of the model is 'variance analysis'. Variance tracking in ICPs offers valuable insights into changes in resource utilization. Variance analysis in standard costing identifies the cost implications of changes in practice, costs and volumes.

Taken together, the two techniques offer the detailed information needed by care managers to achieve and sustain cost-effective health care.

Current costing models in the NHS have no equivalent patient focus. Instead they rely on blocks of resources and activity such as:

- specialties;
- sub-specialties;
- health care related groups (HRGs) and diagnostic related groups (DRGs);
- day cases, in-patients and out-patients;
- diagnostic support;
- rehabilitation.

Traditionally, costs of health care are grouped around specialties. This does not always match the resources taken up by patients. Allocating costs to specialties and then, for example, to HRGs, does not easily enable different components of care to be assigned to patients. In particular, HRGs are currently in-patient focused and need a diagnostic or operating code for classification. Most health care, however, begins with signs and symptoms, making the HRG classification difficult.

A patient focus that matches the ICP approach is essential for meaningful costing.

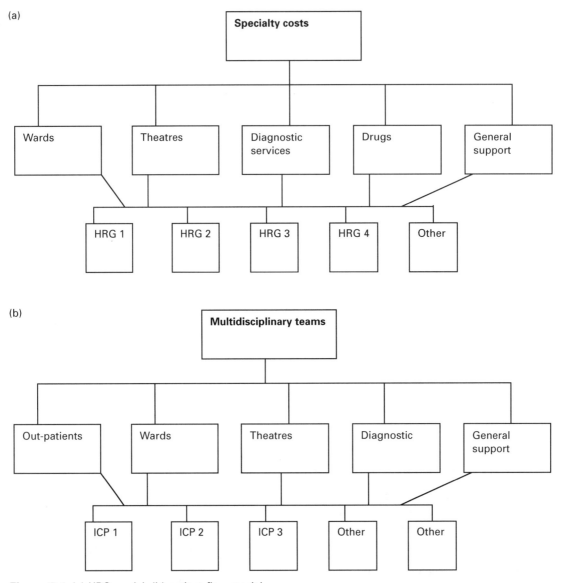

Figure 3.4 (a) HRG model; (b) patient flow model

This avoids the problem where the same condition can have different costs depending on the consultant and the specialty that the patient is assigned to. For example, varicose veins treated in general surgery often carry a different cost to the same treatment provided in a vascular specialty.

Totally absorbed costs used by the NHS form the basis of the national schedule of reference costs. For cost-effective health care, a generic ICP with the same content, standards and outcomes provided by several trusts should have similar total costs – why spend more? In this role, ICPs offer a natural development to HRGs/DRGs.

The ACCA and NPA report proposed an enhanced costing model designed as a shift from the HRG model shown in Figure 3.4(a) to the patient flow model simplified as Figure 3.4(b).

As multidisciplinary teams become more prevalent in health care they tend to form the resource groupings needed for ICPs and they also cut across specialty boundaries. By switching from specialty costs to multidisciplinary costs, as required by ICPs, a better fit of costing to health care can be achieved. However, in the medium term, ICP coverage will not be complete, so both ICP and HRG cost analyses may be needed together.

There are a number of important features of ICP cost models to consider:

- Initially they will be more limited in number than HRGs/DRGs.
- They enable more blocks of resources, such as out-patients, to be apportioned rigorously to patient groups.
- Both models will be needed until ICPs are developed and used more extensively.

Decisions to be made on changes only need costs to be included that can be changed. Hence the indirect costs of fixed assets and high managerial overheads must be excluded. While they are needed as part of a total cost absorption exercise for charging commissioners, they muddy the waters when it comes to ICPs. Health care professionals can agree to improve their cost-effectiveness but decisions about overhead costs are beyond their authority. This leads on to two essential enablers to improve cost-effectiveness with ICPs:

1) Individual ICPs regularly reveal scope to reduce the cost of health care while improving outcomes. However, much of this is a calculation rather than identifying releasable resources. Managers and executive directors need to support health care professionals in extending the range of ICPs across enough activities to achieve a momentum that can:
   - aggregate ICPs and release unneeded direct health care resources; and
   - improve resource utilization enough to enable overheads to be reduced.
2) Improved cost-effectiveness relies extensively on:
   - health care professionals sharing 'real-time' patient and clinical information; and
   - improved scheduling of health care resources to meet patient needs.

Both of these issues require investment in patient and clinical information that differ from current models in the NHS. The NHS strategy 'Information for Health' (Department of Health, 1918), creates an appropriate setting to achieve this. In combination, these enabling efforts can help realize some of the ICP cost gains that have been calculated as often about 30 per cent savings for an individual condition, but are incredibly complex to release. The challenge now is to step up the scale and application of ICPs to impact constructively on the cost base.

Commissioners

Integrating ICPs with standard costing techniques offers scope to support commissioning by primary care groups (PCGs)/local health groups (LHGs). Together with health authorities, they have a great interest in improving cost-effective care. The PCG/LHG perspective is one of matching health care needs to health care provision. With demand constantly outrunning supply and resources, increased cost-effectiveness is one way to help close the gap to some degree. An important emphasis will be in moving health care to the least costly part of the health care continuum whilst continuing to achieve the best outcome.

The immediate challenge for commissioning is to establish how ICPs can:

- be consistently developed;
- become truly integrated;
- be used to bridge the costing issues between health care provided by:
  - hospitals;
  - community hospitals/services;
  - primary care services.

If these issues can be resolved, commissioners can then apply ICPs to improve cost-effectiveness. The split of costs between direct health care and institutional costs has always been awkward due to the fact that health care can develop and improve faster than fixed asset costs can respond. ICPs and their associated costing techniques offer an opportunity to deal with this.

The challenge for commissioners is to design the financial incentives to rapidly improve cost-effectiveness, maybe by developing a parallel allocation policy that splits money into two parts enabling incentives to be designed to match. Considerable reliance will have to be placed on providers for information. It is extremely unlikely that NHS commissioners will ever have the resources needed to set up and operate their own 'managed care' database. Instead, collaboration with providers and access to their data warehouses will be essential to gain the necessary information on:

- benefits and outcomes of each ICP;
- fit to health benefit groups (HBGs);
- rigour of the ICP;
- cost of the ICP;
- variation from the ICP.

With a parallel costing and resource allocation model, this offers a sufficient knowledge base for commissioners to play their part in improving cost-effectiveness. The challenge for commissioners is to devise the financial incentives to facilitate this improvement, using ICPs as the setting to support them.

Conclusions

This chapter has explored how ICPs can act as a framework to facilitate cost-effective health care. The experience of the United States in introducing managed care, however, provides important lessons as to how the drive for cost-efficiency should proceed. A recent review by the ACCA (1999), for example, highlighted considerable anxiety about the expansion of managed care and an extensive reliance on ICPs. Pathways are mainly used by health maintenance organizations in the USA and are seen as a focus for managing costs rather than managing care.

Fortunately, the primary purpose of ICPs in the UK has been to improve both the quality and outcome of health care. Their role in improving cost-effectiveness can therefore be seen as crucial in terms of balancing the equation of quality and cost.

References

ACCA (1999) *Some directions for the NHS from New England, USA – Report on an ACCA study tour*. London, Association of Chartered Certified Accountants.

ACCA and NPA (1999) *Managing Care Pathways*. London, Association of Chartered Certified Accountants and National Pathways Association.

Department of Health (1998) *Information for Health*. London.

ICPs: a vehicle to deliver clinical governance

Denise Kitchiner

Introduction

The concept of clinical governance (Scally and Donaldson, 1998) is an extension of a number of initiatives introduced into the NHS in recent years. These include clinical audit (de Lacey, 1992), the use of multidisciplinary guidelines (Delamothe, 1994; Thomson et al., 1995) and evidence-based practice (Sackett et al., 1995), continuous quality improvement, clinical effectiveness, patient-focused care and clinical risk management. Many of these initiatives have important theoretical benefits but, at a practical level, they have been difficult to embed into routine patient care. Clinical governance focuses on a comprehensive programme of continuous quality improvement for which senior clinicians and managers are directly responsible. It includes processes for monitoring care and external review, policies for managing risk and clear lines of responsibility and accountability. It has moved the emphasis from the cost of health care to the quality of clinical practice. For this reason it should be welcomed by clinicians, but the practical problem of translating the concept into a working reality remains. Mechanisms need to be in place to facilitate the incorporation of these principles into routine clinical practice. ICPs provide a practical tool to monitor and improve patient care, thereby enabling clinicians to achieve the targets set by the clinical governance agenda.

Delivering a quality service

ICPs support the delivery of a quality service by helping us to:

- complete the audit cycle;
- manage change;
- increase the body of knowledge where little evidence exists;
- manage clinical risk; and
- incorporate guidelines into everyday practice.

Completing the audit cycle

It remains extremely difficult to conduct a comprehensive multidisciplinary audit as part of routine clinical practice. Problems include the retrospective evaluation of incomplete information and the extra documentation required to collect the data needed for a prospective audit. It is often difficult to evaluate whether audit changes clinical practice and whether any change is sustained after the audit project is completed. Involvement of all members of the multidisciplinary team may also be hard to achieve. Nevertheless, the systematic evaluation of clinical practice is an integral part of patient care. This should include the development and implementation of clinical standards or guidelines and the continuous evaluation of the process and outcome of care against these standards. There must also be a mechanism to improve clinical practice as a result of this process.

A well-organized ICP programme can provide continuous audit, including re-evaluation of changes in clinical practice. In doing this, it fulfils many of the requirements of clinical governance. A retrospective case-note review of patients who have recently been treated provides an accurate assessment of current practice and this can be compared with recognized guidelines and evidence-based practice. Involvement of members of the multidisciplinary team also ensures that the ICP reflects locally agreed best practice. Current clinical practice is then continuously evaluated by documenting and analysing variations from these standards as defined by the ICP. Analysis of variations from the ICP is a powerful audit tool as all aspects of patient care are reviewed continuously and revised. In order to do this, it is necessary to have a method of collecting information on variations from the ICP together with the cause and the action taken. Positive variation occurs when goals are achieved more quickly than expected, and negative variation indicates goals that are not met on time, in the correct sequence or simply not achieved. An adverse outcome would also be considered a negative variation. The causes may be avoidable if inefficiencies have occurred, or unavoidable if they are due to the individual patient's condition or response to treatment.

Analysis of variations provides accurate information on the frequency and the cause of variations in patient care. This allows the multidisciplinary team to develop solutions to unnecessary variations in clinical practice (Kitchiner and Pozzi, 1999). The analysis encourages members of the team to adhere to the guidelines and standards set by the ICP, or justify the reason for any variations. This helps to improve clinical outcomes and the quality of patient care, by reducing avoidable variation in the clinical process (Chassin, 1996).

Documentation and analysis of variations also highlights trends. It can identify problems that may not have been noticed previously. If an aspect of care has changed, the impact of this change can be evaluated. Analysis of variations from the ICP also provides valuable information on the clinical outcomes in all patients.

ICPs were introduced to the Cardiac Unit at the Royal Liverpool Children's Hospital in July 1994. They were developed for patients undergoing cardiac surgery for atrial septal defect, ventricular septal defect, Fallot's tetralogy, aortic coarctation and partial and complete atrioventricular septal defect. More recently other pathways have been developed for patients undergoing cardiac catheterization, a pre-operative pathway for all patients, an analgesia pathway for all patients after cardiac surgery and pathways for the use of streptokinase and alteplase for vascular obstruction. Due to the introduction of these ICPs a number of aspects of care are constantly monitored. These include analgesia

after surgery, duration of ventilation and length of stay in intensive care following cardiac surgery, the timing of temporary pacing wire removal and the length of stay after cardiac surgery. This programme has been the main method of ongoing clinical audit in the directorate since 1994.

Identification of a variation is also useful in individual patient care. It allows the multidisciplinary team to identify the specific needs of each patient in the most effective and efficient way. If a patient deviates from the ICP, the team is given an early warning that the patient is not doing as well as expected. This allows the cause to be identified and treated.

Improvements in the quality of care are rapidly achieved by continuously re-defining the ICPs to reflect current best practice. ICPs are dynamic documents. Improvements in practice and specific recommendations or guidelines can be introduced by revising the ICP. These changes can be implemented immediately and used in the care of all subsequent patients. Changes in practice are re-evaluated, resulting in continuous improvement in the quality of care provided. This facilitates the inclusion of multidisciplinary audit and continuous quality improvement into routine clinical care.

Managing change

Many of the initiatives introduced into the NHS over the last ten years have required changes in practice. Most were aimed at an efficient use of limited resources, but were often perceived by clinicians as limiting clinical freedom in order to cut costs. The introduction of the clinical governance agenda has moved the emphasis from the cost of health care, to a process of managing clinical care in order to improve quality within the resources available. This has given clinicians the opportunity to control and direct the change rather than managers. However, clinicians still need tools to bring about that change and ICPs encourage changes that are clinically led rather than management driven.

At the Royal Liverpool Children's NHS Trust, ICPs have been used to identify areas where changes were needed and to bring about that improvement. Post-operative analgesia, for example, has been found to be a problem. Information obtained from the retrospective analysis indicated that post-operative analgesia was not being given regularly on the first two post-operative days. Review of the number of doses of analgesia actually given suggested that this was likely to have been suboptimal for adequate analgesia. Assessing the degree of pain is difficult in infants and young children. Therefore a comprehensive audit of post-operative analgesia resulted in the development of therapeutic guidelines that have been incorporated into the ICP. The adequacy of post-operative analgesia was subsequently evaluated in all patients who were on an ICP after operation. The number of patients receiving inadequate post-operative analgesia has decreased significantly.

Increasing the body of knowledge where little evidence exists

Evidence-based clinical practice encourages clinicians to make their decisions on information that indicates which forms of therapy or management are most effective. Unfortunately many aspects of our clinical practice are not based on sound scientific evidence. It is also not always certain that evidence can be transferred from the clinical situation where it was collected to that which applies in another institution. It is therefore important to collect information locally to support practice in that specific clinical setting.

After cardiac surgery, many patients have temporary pacing wires that are removed before discharge. There is great variability in the timing of pacing wire removal. Reviewing the literature was no help as there was no evidence as to the optimum timing for this procedure. A randomized trial is potentially unethical as early removal carries a theoretical risk of bleeding and cardiac tamponade. At the Royal Liverpool Children's NHS Trust we now remove the wires on the fourth post-operative day if the patient is in sinus rhythm. Analysis of the outcome in patients over the last four years has shown that this is a safe procedure with no complications related to removal of wires a day earlier than previously. It has also allowed a number of patients to be discharged a day earlier than would otherwise have been the case.

Some patients have additional clinical conditions that may cause variations from the ICP. It is important to evaluate whether they need a different ICP because the combination of conditions results in a different clinical course. The way to do this is to look at the variations from the ICP. In a study of patients following cardiac surgery at the Royal Liverpool Children's NHS Trust, patients with Down's syndrome were compared with other patients. Those with Down's syndrome who underwent repair of an atrial or ventricular septal defect did not have longer duration of ventilation, length of intensive care stay or time in hospital after operation. This information indicated that it was not necessary to write a separate ICP for these patients and that their management should be no different from those without Down's syndrome.

Managing clinical risk

Clinical risk management is an important aspect of clinical governance.[1] Significant untoward events are closely related to variations in clinical practice. These may occur because of lack of awareness of, or compliance with, recognized clinical guidelines. The reoccurrence of errors that lead to a serious risk for patients or staff is also sometimes the cause. ICPs can be used to identify areas of clinical risk. At the time when the ICP is being developed, case-note review and discussion with the multidisciplinary team may identify areas of potential risk. Incorporation of generally accepted guidelines and evidence-based practice into the ICP also helps to reduce risk. Potential risks can be identified and procedures established to minimize them. By including these in the ICP, changes in practice can rapidly be communicated to all members of the multidisciplinary team. As the ICP remains in the patient's record, it facilitates communication and documentation of the care needed and the care provided. It also encourages adherence to guidelines.

Analysis of variations from the ICP can also be used to monitor areas of potential risk. Poor documentation can fail to indicate whether a guideline has been followed. This can readily be addressed by the introduction of the ICP. Another aspect of risk management is the prevention of recurrence of untoward events. ICPs can include guidelines that ensure all health professionals are aware of potential risks and take appropriate action to prevent them from occurring.

Incorporating guidelines into everyday practice

Clinical effectiveness involves not only the development of evidence-based guidelines, but their use in clinical practice. Poor quality health care is frequently associated with unjustifiable variations in clinical practice and standardization of clinical practice has been shown to improve outcomes (O'Connor et al., 1996). Implementation of clinical guidelines remains difficult to achieve (Thomson, 1995). Even when clinicians agree to guidelines, they do not necessarily follow them (Lomas et al., 1989) and many more guidelines are written than are used in routine patient care. The reasons for this are complex, but include lack of awareness or acceptance of nationally developed guidelines, and arbitrary variations in clinical practice. Many of the current methods used to develop guidelines include the 'top-down' approach, with guidelines being developed by expert panels. This fails to take into consideration the views of the many professional groups involved in a patient's care.

The use of clinical practice guidelines based on the best available evidence has generally been welcomed, but implementation requires specific action at a local level. The use of ICPs facilitates the implementation of multidisciplinary guidelines into routine clinical practice. ICPs set locally agreed standards that are based on evidence or on observation data where more robust evidence is not available. These standards or guidelines are used to evaluate our clinical practice. Analysis of variations from the guidelines allows a continuous evaluation of the effectiveness of clinical practice.

The development of the ICP gives the multidisciplinary team an ideal opportunity to critically evaluate current practice. It encourages clinicians to review evidence-based guidelines and include them in the ICP. Adherence to guidelines is facilitated as the ICP forms part of the patient's record, and is available for review when clinical decisions are being made. Compliance is further encouraged as the guidelines are locally agreed, and deviations must be documented and clinically justified by stating the reason for the variation from the accepted standard. Analysis of the causes of variation from the ICP provides valuable information which can be used to evaluate clinical practice and the reasons for deviation from the ICP. It also allows clinicians to audit the effectiveness of national guidelines at a local level, and to collect observational evidence when randomized trials are impractical or unjustified.

Conclusions

Some clinicians believe that the ICPs, protocols and guidelines over-emphasize the clinical condition at the expense of individual patient care. In practice, we have found the opposite appears to be the case. ICPs provide patient-focused care as they constantly monitor the quality of the care provided. In addition, deviations from the ICP identify complications early. The plan of care is clearly defined and shared with the patient/carer. In some instances patients have been involved in the development and evaluation of the ICP. Discharge planning is also facilitated as the median length of stay for the particular condition is defined. As Dowsey et al. (1999) and Rossiter et al. (1998) have shown, ICPs reduce the length of stay, without an increase in complications or unscheduled re-attendance. Dowsey and colleagues have also shown that when they introduced ICPs for hip and knee joint arthroplasty better patient outcomes were achieved.

Through the use of ICPs, it has been possible to quantify inefficiencies and this facilitates the development of solutions to potentially avoidable problems and delays. It also provides detailed information on patient outcomes and allows development of locally agreed guidelines based on observational data.

ICPs require time and effort on the part of the multidisciplinary team to develop and maintain. Time is also needed to educate staff and analyse the variation from the ICP. However, the systematic evaluation of clinical practice is becoming essential. The requirements of clinical governance mean that the multidisciplinary team will need to have the tools to critically examine the outcomes of the services that they provide. ICPs provide a continuous cycle of evaluation and improvement in clinical practice. They are becoming recognized as a practical tool to incorporate clinical effectiveness and clinical governance into routine patient care.

References

Chassin, M.R. (1996) Quality of Health Care. Part 3: Improving the Quality of Care. *New England Journal of Medicine*, 335, 1060–3.

Delamothe, T. (1994) Wanted: guidelines that doctors will follow. *British Medical Journal*, 307, 218.

Dowsey, M., Kilgour, M., Santamaria, N. and Choong, P.F.M. (1999) A prospective study of clinical pathways in hip and knee arthroplasty. *Medical Journal of Australia*, 170, 56–60.

Kitchiner, D. and Pozzi, M. (1999) Integrated Care Pathways – a tool for the continuous evaluation of clinical practice. *Cardiology News*, 2, 6–7.

de Lacey, G. (1992) What is audit? Why should we be doing it? *Hospital Update*, 22, 458–66.

Lomas, J., Amderson, G.M., Dominick-Pierre, K., Vayda, E., Enkin, M.W. and Hannah, W.J. (1989) Do practice guidelines guide practice? The effect of a consensus statement on the practice of physicians. *New England Journal of Medicine*, 321, 1306–11.

O'Connor, G.T., Plume, S.K., Olmstead, E.M., Morton, J.R., Maloney, C.T., Nugent, W.C., Hernandez, F., Clough, R., Leavitt, B.J., Coffin, L.H., Marrin, C.A., Wennberg, D., Birkmeyer, J.D., Charlsworth, D.C., Malenka, D.J., Quinton, H.B. and Kasper, J.F. (1996) A regional intervention to improve the hospital mortality associated with coronary artery bypass graft surgery. *Journal of the American Medical Association*, 275, 841–6.

Rossiter, D.A., Edmondson, A., Al-Shahi, R. and Thompson, A.J. (1998) Integrated care pathways in multiple sclerosis rehabilitation: completing the audit cycle. *Multiple Sclerosis*, 4, 85–9.

Sackett, D.L., Rosenberg, W.M.C., Gray, J.A.M., Haynes, R.B. and Richardson, W.S. (1995) Evidence based medicine: what it is and what it isn't. *British Medical Journal*, 312, 71–2.

Scally, G. and Donaldson, L.J. (1998) Clinical governance and the drive for quality improvement in the new NHS in England. *British Medical Journal*, 317, 61–5.

Thomson, R., Lavender, M. and Madhok, R. (1995) How to ensure that guidelines are effective. *British Medical Journal*, 311, 237–42.

Part Three

HOW TO INTRODUCE INTEGRATED CARE PATHWAYS

5

Getting started

Sue Middleton and Adrian Roberts

Summary

- A strategic approach: a vision of the future
- Role of the facilitator
- Stages of ICP development

Introduction

Between September 1995 and March 1997, the VFM Unit (NHS Wales), the Clinical Resource Utilisation Group (Welsh Office) undertook a major project designed to understand the nature of ICP activity in the UK. The project aimed to identify the critical success factors and potential barriers to the adoption of ICPs and to develop a 'framework' or structured approach to support successful implementation.

By completion, the project team had collated and taken into consideration the views of over 700 clinical, managerial and operational staff involved in the design and use of ICPs. A key result of the project was the identification of five distinct and sequential stages used by organizations with evidence of successful programmes of ICP activity. These stages were defined as:

1. Awareness raising and gaining commitment.
2. Putting systems into place.
3. Documentation.
4. Implementation.
5. Evaluation.

This chapter focuses on *Stage 1* Awareness raising and gaining commitment, and *Stage 2* Putting systems into place, to provide practical information on **how to get started with ICPs**.

Awareness raising and gaining commitment

A strategic approach: a vision of the future

The successful development and application of ICPs requires a shared understanding of what the organization is seeking to achieve. The commitment of senior management and clinical staff is essential and entails creating a 'vision' of the future, to which all staff can subscribe. This helps to ensure that everybody is working towards a set of common strategic aims that can be developed into a framework for service delivery.

As a change management tool, ICPs should be included as an integral component in the organization's business and quality strategies and form part of any system developed to address clinical governance. The use of ICPs can be aligned to suit organizational objectives and as a 'building block' in the strategic plan to manage the quality of patient care, the flow of patients through the organization, evidence-based health care, audit and clinical risk.

In practice, the 'vision' of an organization tends to build up over time. However, a lead is provided for the NHS by the periodic publication of government papers and other related documents that outline strategy for a defined period of time. For example, the recent NHS Wales white paper reinforced a vision set out for the NHS ten years earlier and is based on the following values (NHS Wales, 1998b):

- The NHS should be health gain focused, seeking to reduce both the number of premature deaths in Wales and to improve the quality of life.
- It should be people-centred, managing its services for the benefit of patients and informed by patients' views.
- The service should be resource effective.

In addition, a set of 'key objectives' were outlined to support this vision:

- to remove obstacles to integrated care;
- to develop local responsiveness to take advantage of the greatly enhanced prospects for providing care in, and close to, patients' homes;

- to reduce health variations across Wales and tackle inequalities in health and in access to health care;
- to better align responsibilities for clinical and financial decisions within local settings which are best able to deliver integrated programmes of care;
- to exploit modern technology to the full to provide better information to people and their local GPs so that both may make better informed choices about care;
- to improve efficiency at all levels within and between organizations and their individual members of staff;
- to enhance the quality of care, starting with good quality research and development, which embraces clinical effectiveness and includes organizational performance measured, in part, by programmes of continuous benchmarking, and
- to make the continuous training and development of staff at all levels and in all sectors a priority.

For organizations, or indeed individual directorates and departments, seeking to clarify their vision of the future they will realistically need to take account of the prevailing agenda. To be specific, however, it can be helpful to consider the following questions:

- What are we trying to achieve (i.e. what are our objectives as an organization, directorate, department)?
- What is the best way of achieving these objectives?
- What is the best way of communicating our plans throughout the organization?
- How do we ensure the commitment of all our staff?

Expressing their 'vision' in this manner allows organizations to identify both potential barriers to change and those who are supportive of change. This is particularly important in the development of ICPs as a strong medical lead is essential with a motivated and influential consultant required to head each 'project'. Early identification of support can also be helpful in encouraging more reluctant peers to become involved.

Reasons for developing ICPs

Within the organizational vision, it is important to reinforce the aims of ICPs in line with

organizational objectives. Three main reasons have been identified for the development of ICPs (VFM Unit, 1997). These are:

(1) To improve the quality of patient care through consistent management by:
- encouraging patient involvement;
- identifying and measuring improvements/outcomes in patient care.
(2) To promote the efficient use of resources without compromising the quality of patient care delivery by:
- reducing unnecessary documentation;
- facilitating a plan of care from pre-admission assessment to discharge (for acute care) and improving links with and between community services.
(3) To increase collaboration between disciplines/professionals/agencies to ensure continuity of patient care by:
- reducing unnecessary variations in the management of patient care, and documenting variations from the predicted plan of care;
- ensuring that no critical aspect(s) of care are forgotten and that all interventions are planned appropriately and are performed on time;
- providing a framework for effective clinical audit;
- serving as an educational and training tool including orientation of new/bank staff or staff on short rotation.

A 'personal vision' for ICPs:

Each ICP will:

- follow the patient
- cross professional and organizational boundaries
- be based on available evidence or consensus of best practice
- form a single record of care
- be audited
- build on each other, e.g. acute/rehab/terminal care.

The role of the ICP facilitator

A common concern expressed by clinicians prior to the development of ICPs relates to the pressure placed on already busy staff and limited resources by yet another initiative, which initially at least requires some time to be spent away from direct patient care. These concerns can be addressed, in part, by the appointment of a dedicated ICP facilitator. The skills and ability of the facilitator are likely to be key factors in the success or otherwise of the ICP programme (Stephens, 1997, p.156).

The facilitator's role will be to:

- raise awareness of ICP activity;
- provide initial training, ongoing education and support;
- act as a 'link' between all professional groups involved;
- set up and 'manage' individual ICP 'projects';
- attend and facilitate ICP development meetings;
- prepare ICP documentation;
- provide ongoing evaluation, feedback and review.

ICP facilitator: skills checklist (Stephens, 1997, p.157)

1. Presentation and training ☐
2. Communication and negotiation ☐
3. Project management/change management ☐
4. Team building and group facilitation ☐
5. Computer literate/IT skills ☐
6. Ability to motivate/lead as appropriate ☐
7. Ability to work to tight deadlines under pressure ☐
8. Sound knowledge of ICPs and related initiatives ☐
9. Confidence, credibility and self-motivation ☐

Awareness raising sessions and encouraging staff involvement
A key task for the ICP facilitator will be to run a series of 'awareness sessions' aimed at encouraging staff involvement in the design and implementation of ICPs. It is important that all staff to be involved are consulted prior to beginning a programme of development.

The awareness sessions provide an opportunity for staff to air any concerns or reservations they have about the ICP approach. The key here is to be honest and to try to answer all questions and any anxieties that may

surface and to tackle any misconceptions that may be held about ICPs.

The sessions also allow staff to outline any frustrations they experience in dealing with particular patient groups and to discuss how ICPs can help to minimize them. This is helpful in managing staff expectations as to what ICPs can and cannot do. Some NHS trusts have approached this issue by asking staff what information they require from the ICP approach and focusing on their responses.

Putting systems into place

Selecting your patient group(s)

The success of your ICP will often depend on selecting an appropriate patient group(s). Initially, in order to gain confidence and experience, the criteria outlined below can help guide your selection.

Common condition (high percentage of patients)
The majority of the workload of most clinical teams and individual specialties is made up of a small number of clinical conditions and interventions. By selecting these conditions you will be concentrating on the client groups that have the biggest impact on your organization, allowing these patients to be managed more efficiently and releasing more time to be spent

Table 5.1 Common reasons for contact

Clinical team/specialty	Common reason for contact
Surgical ward	Hernia repair
Cardiac surgical ward	Coronary artery by-pass graft
Medical ward	Acute and chronic chest infection
Urology ward	TURP
Children's ward	Febrile convulsions
Orthopaedic department	Fractured neck of femur*
A&E department	Chest pain
Community nurses	Leg ulcers
Health visitors	Immunization
Midwives	Monitoring
General practitioners	Infections
Practice nurses	Dressings
Physiotherapists	Assessment
Dieticians	Advice
Occupational therapists	Assessment

*Fractured neck of femur is the most popular ICP topic within acute services according to a survey carried out by the National Pathways Association (1998).

on the less common, often more complex and unpredictable patients.

Simple condition (i.e. not multi-pathology)
Concentrating on 'simple' conditions with a defined sequence of events and a clear start and end point can help to demonstrate 'quick wins' and early success which is often useful in motivating more reluctant peers to become involved in ICP development. However, a basic pathway can potentially be designed for all conditions by recognizing the three aspects of all care planning regardless of diagnosis or setting (NHS Wales, 1998a):

- physical and mental assessment of the patient;
- patient education on their disease, medication and lifestyle; and
- milestones to be reached before discharge.

Problem areas
ICPs can be developed to address specific problem areas, e.g. where audit results suggest there is room for improvements in performance or if a high number of complaints are received about a particular aspect of care.

Staff expressed preferences
Focusing on a staff expressed preference helps to ensure the commitment of all professionals involved in the design and implementation of the ICP.

There are a number of other valid reasons for developing an ICP, often relating to issues that are high on the current agenda. These reasons often link with the criteria outlined above and can be defined as follows.

Monitoring and comparing clinical outcomes
Outcome measures are beginning to be used to compare performance, both between different organizations and different clinicians. A common practice in the United States, the emphasis in the UK has until recently been placed upon measuring waiting times for specific surgical interventions or triage time within accident and emergency departments.

There have, however, been a number of moves towards more 'meaningful' and comprehensive data collection and comparison covering length of stay, cost per case, re-admission rates, mortality, morbidity and infection rates. The new NHS Performance Assessment Framework, for example, provides a structure for reviewing NHS performance against outcomes of importance to patients and the public (NHS Executive, 1999, p.10), focusing on:

- population group, for example, geographic area, ethnic minority or social class;
- **condition/patient group, for example, coronary heart disease, asthma and chronic respiratory disease, children**;
- service organization, for example health authority, NHS trust or PCG.

When performance comparisons of this type are presented 'in isolation' or in 'league tables' it is often easy to explain away areas of weak performance (*'we are different', 'we have a more complicated case mix', 'we have an older and poorer population'*). All of these responses may be valid but by placing this performance information within the ICP approach and by beginning a critical appraisal of our current practice we can start to explore and resolve the reasons why patients do not always proceed as expected.

ICPs can also be developed where there are substantial variations in practice and outcomes between individual clinicians within the same organization.

Meeting health gain targets
National Service Frameworks will set national standards and define service models for a specific service or care group, put in programmes to support implementation and establish performance measures against which progress within an agreed timescale will be measured (NHS Executive, 1999, p.7).

It may be appropriate to choose these patient groups for ICP development, using the ICP as a vehicle to incorporate the information contained in the frameworks into every-day practice.

Similarly, The Welsh Office published a set of fifteen **health gain targets** for Wales in June 1997 (DGM (97) 50). The targets cover:

- lung cancer
- breast cancer
- cervical cancer
- heart disease
- strokes
- accidents

- suicides
- low birth weight
- back pain
- arthritis
- mental health
- smoking
- consumption of fruit and vegetables
- consumption of alcohol
- dental caries

This set of targets is not a comprehensive list of conditions nor a list of priorities but does represent, together with targets for 'children's health and well being' (Welsh Office, 1997), the 'best available' set of indicators and targets for overall improvement of health and well-being in Wales (Welsh Office, 1998). In addition, each health authority area is to develop a series of health improvement programmes, outlining how these targets will be met. Again, it may be appropriate to consider the use of ICPs to support this process.

The availability of evidence/guidelines
In terms of clinical effectiveness, it is perhaps simpler in the early stages of ICP development to choose topics which have robust evidence or clear guidelines available for diagnosing, assessing or managing the patient group. The availability of evidence to support clinical practice and decision making together with the existence of 'nationally' agreed guidelines helps to facilitate local consensus between professional colleagues. Examples of these topics include myocardial infarction and asthma.

Managing clinical risk
Those clients presenting with a higher than average clinical risk may comprise the majority of patients cared for by some clinical teams. Alternatively, for many clinical teams, less common or rare conditions may provide the highest risk due to the limited experience staff may have in relation to these patients. For example, to retain the skills necessary to perform cardiac massage, it is necessary to practice the technique at least once every twelve months.

The use of ICPs in these situations helps to ensure that all staff are aware of the necessary interventions required for management of the case type in question.

Agreeing the scope of the ICP
Defining the scope of the ICP involves establishing where each patient enters and ultimately leaves the sphere of control of the pathway. In essence, this means agreeing a start point (e.g. GP consultation, pre-admission clinic, admission, etc.) an end point (transfer from A&E, discharge, home visit(s) in the community, etc.) and the boundaries of the pathway. For ICPs that cross organizational boundaries it is probably simpler for each organization to develop their own section of the pathway before 'building' it into a completed document. The decisions concerning the scope of the ICP will influence who will be involved in the development of the pathway and the defined objective(s) of the care to be provided.

Managing paediatric asthma in A&E

Start point: Arrival and triage at A&E

End point: Discharge home/transfer to children's ward

Boundaries: Accident and emergency department

An ICP of this nature can be seen as a 'mini-pathway' which can be used as a 'building-block' for further development. The start point, end point and boundaries of the pathway are fluid. The ICP could be extended to include GPs, the primary health care team and paramedics (prior to admission), the children's ward (after transfer) and GPs and the primary health care team (following discharge).

The development team
ICPs aim to improve communication between the members of a clinical team. As such, the development team needs to include a representative sample of *all* the professionals involved in providing care for the chosen patient group. For many, the multidisciplinary debate generated by the development team is the most valuable element of ICP development, helping to break down any barriers that may exist and fostering closer working relationships. Even clinical teams that have spent a considerable amount of time working together may be surprised at how much they learn about their fellow professionals' input into the care cycle.

Whenever possible, dedicated time and support should be set aside for development team meetings.

Sample development team – suspected myocardial infarction ICP

Medical staff, A&E and CCU
Nursing staff, A&E and CCU
Receptionist A&E
CCU clerk
Pharmacy
Pathology staff
ECG technician
Paramedical staff
Portering staff

Key: A&E = accident and emergency; CCU = coronary care unit; ECG = electrocardiograph

---

Defining the desired objective(s) of care

The first step for the development team is to define the desired objective(s) of care for the chosen patient group. Objectives can relate to:

- patient outcomes
- patient satisfaction
- service quality
- cost effectiveness and efficiency.

Expressing the desired outcome(s) of care as SMART goals helps to ensure that they are both meaningful and measurable:

SPECIFIC: not capable of misinterpretation

MEASURABLE: possible to tell if they have been achieved or not

ACTION ORIENTED: probably ending with 'in order to achieve . . . . .'

REALISTIC achievable using the available resources

TIME RELATED with a target date for completion.

Defining desired outcome(s) is important, as each outcome will help to confirm the scope of the ICP and can also be used to provide a 'health check' of both current practice and of the ICP following implementation. Objective

setting is also a useful tool in terms of maintaining commitment, with clinical staff playing an active role in defining the standard(s) of care they wish their patients to receive.

Desired objectives can be informed by available evidence, clinical audit and benchmarking data, accreditation standards, health-gain targets, national service frameworks, etc.

Sample SMART objectives

'100 per cent of all patients presenting with an MI will receive thrombolysis (taking into account contra-indications) within 30 minutes of arriving through the door, in order to comply with available evidence as to best quality of care.'
'100 per cent of all patients presenting with symptoms of leg ulcer referred to appropriate professional within one week and management of ulcer commenced in order to achieve anticipated clinical outcome.'

Mapping the current process of care

The next stage for the development team is to 'process map' the care *currently* provided to the chosen patient group. A process map is essentially a picture of the activities or tasks that over time deliver a product, outcome or achieves a desired condition. The map helps to define:

- the sequence of steps and activities performed;
- specific responsibilities for these steps and activities;
- areas that lie 'outside' the process but have an impact on it;
- the relationships that exist between the different professionals in the process;
- potential problem areas ('failure points') and opportunities for improvements in current practice.

The initial process map needs to be kept simple ('high-level'), including the 6–10 key elements used to deliver care to your chosen patient group. A case-note review of the last 10–20 patients will help to complete this map (for example, Figure 5.2) which is used as a basis for the more detailed mapping required to inform the ICP document.

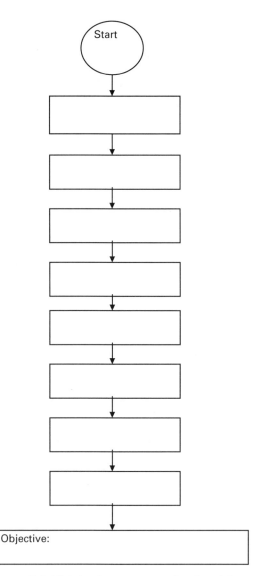

Figure 5.1 High-level process mapping template

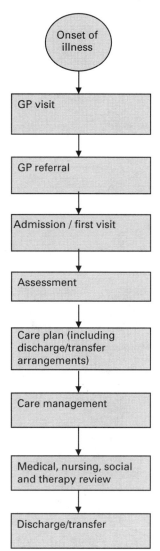

Figure 5.2 Sub-acute admission to community hospital/intermediate services: high-level process map

More detailed process mapping

The key to successful process mapping is to start simple before becoming steadily more complex. By using the 'high-level' map as a template, the development team can map each of the identified 6–10 elements in more detail to gain a comprehensive overview of the whole process (For example, Figure 5.3). Some organizations have found it helpful to have each 'individual' profession map their own

input into care before assembling the final process map.

In order to ensure that the more detailed maps remain focused it is important to define the desired objective(s) and agree the scope for **each additional** map drawn by the development team. As you will now be including more than 6–10 elements in your map, it is best, however, to switch to a horizontal format. A standard format is to link four or five elements in rows across the page using the

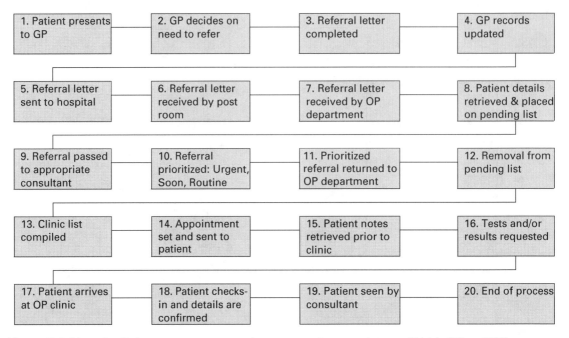

Figure 5.3 More detailed process map – arranging an outpatient appointment (Welsh Office, 1999)

connector symbol (Figure 5.4) to join pages where necessary.

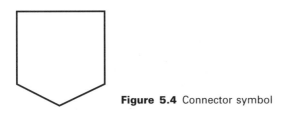

Figure 5.4 Connector symbol

The value of process mapping

Process maps are important because they help the development team define *what actually happens* when care is provided to the chosen patient group rather than what is supposed to happen. This allows the team to evaluate their current practice against the clinical evidence base and to ask questions about the appropriateness of particular activities, tasks and investigations. If any failure points or opportunities for improvement are identified, appropriate changes in practice can be agreed and included in the final pathway. In this context, ICPs can be

seen as a logical way of incorporating clinical effectiveness into routine practice.

The completed multidisciplinary maps also establish a link between the process (i.e. what happens) and outcome (i.e. what is achieved). They can be used to support a clinical bench-marking exercise and to achieve a 'consensus' as to what constitutes best practice. If the desired outcome is completely 'missed' by the current practice the maps also act as a starting point for a more drastic redesign of the process. Further guidance on clinical bench-marking can be found in **Chapter 10.**

Moving from the process map to the ICP document

At this stage, the development team can begin to think how the process mapping information can be translated into the ICP document. By following the stages of development outlined in this chapter, the team should have a set of process maps which 'break' the patient's journey into a series of manageable stages. In order to define the information to be included in the final ICP document, the next step for the team is to examine the maps and identify:

- the criteria for entrance to and exit from each step in the process and/or stage in the patient's journey;
- the assessment tools to be used;
- decision points within the process;
- the investigations and interventions to be performed and who is the most appropriate professional to perform them;
- criteria for referral to other professionals and agencies;
- milestones and outcome measures;
- any guidelines or protocols to be included;
- patient information;
- staff education and training;
- monitoring arrangements.

Conclusion

The information gathered in the processes of *'awareness raising and gaining commitment'* and *'putting systems into place'* is essential for the development of the chosen ICP(s). **Chapter 6, Documentation**, considers how this information is used to design an ICP.

References

NHS Executive (1999) *The NHS Performance Assessment Framework*. Leeds, NHS Executive.

NHS Wales (1998a) *Introduction to clinical pathways*. Cardiff, Welsh Office.

NHS Wales (1998b) *Putting Patients First*. Cardiff, Welsh Office.

Stephens, Rosie (1997) *Setting up pathways in mental health*. In Wilson, Jo (ed.), *Integrated Care Management: The Path to Success*. Oxford, Butterworth–Heinemann.

VFM Unit (1997) *An introduction to Clinical Pathways*. Wrexham, VFM Unit.

Welsh Office (1997) *The Health of Children in Wales*. Cardiff, Welsh Office.

Welsh Office (1998) *Better Health Better Wales*. Cardiff, Welsh Office.

Welsh Office (1999) *An introduction to clinical process redesign*. Cardiff, Welsh Office.

6

Documentation

Sue Middleton and Adrian Roberts

Background

The way that the information collected during the getting started phase of ICP development is formalized into the pathway document will have an impact on its success, particularly in terms of maintaining compliance from the staff who will use it. There are no set rules as to how an ICP should appear on paper and methods of documentation will be influenced both by skills and experience and the nature of the client group involved. However, a consensus has emerged to suggest that ICP documentation *should* be:

- sequential, including a time-frame and clear indicators of how effectively the client moves along their journey;
- written in plain language, avoiding abbreviations if possible unless they have been agreed by the multidisciplinary team;
- presented on A4 paper, portrait not landscape, using 10pt font as minimum.

Process or outcome?

Whether the ICP document is process or outcome based depends on the skills and experience of the staff who will use it. *Process-*

Following surgery, it is important to 'observe' the wound site to ensure that healing has begun and that there are no signs of infection.
A typical example of process-based documentation is:
check wound   ✔ (signature)

based documentation is preferred when the ICP is needed as a checklist or an aide-memoir within those clinical areas with a high turnover of staff or where 'bank' staff are used, when there is a new intake of junior house officers or when patients are cared for in an 'outlying' environment if beds are in short supply.

Many professionals, however, may feel that simply listing a series of processes within the ICP document discourages the health care worker from thinking outside of these parameters. If this is the case, then important symptoms may be missed if the patient veers away from the pathway.

The example of process-based documentation highlighted above ensures that the wound is checked, but realistically what does this mean? Just because the wound has been checked does not necessarily mean that it has begun to heal. In addition, the variation against this statement would be 'the wound has not been checked' which again tells us nothing of the patient's condition.

It is in this kind of situation that outcome-based documentation should be used.

wound dry   ✔ (signature)

This statement anticipates that normal healing of a surgical wound will take place, providing us with valuable information about the patient's condition. In addition, the variation would be that the wound has not begun to heal and therefore remedial action is required.

Most ICPs will include a mixture of *process-*based (the tasks that we need to perform) and *outcome*-based (milestones the patient needs to reach to progress along the pathway) documentation.

ICPs as the legal record of care

ICPs are condition specific, with the content defined by the experience, knowledge and skills of staff working in a particular area. Full compliance with an ICP should ensure that the optimum level of relevant information is gathered and recorded and nothing pertinent is missed, providing the opportunity to introduce a single legal record of care.

However, some disciplines may wish to continue to keep their own records separately from the information included in the pathway. This is particularly important for those professionals who see patients at different times and in different places from where the ICP document is held. If this is the case, it can be suggested that the second set of notes contain condensed information which can be expanded upon as necessary when access to the ICP document is possible.

Introduction of a single record of care does require sensitive and careful handling. A full assessment of any perceived legal implications and other staff concerns should be undertaken prior to any move of this nature.

Flexibility

ICP documents are intended to be flexible, changes are inevitable and are to be encouraged to avoid current practice becoming 'entrenched' as the norm. Review of the documentation in use should occur on an annual basis as a minimum, or if one or more of the following changes occur:

- new evidence becomes available and is accepted by the multidisciplinary team;
- there is a change in the environment or location where care is provided;
- review of the pathway identifies a trend of avoidable variations;
- length of stay reduces as a result of using the ICP;
- lack of compliance with the ICP – this may be caused by a design fault, duplication of information or poor clarification of roles and responsibilities;
- there is a change in skill mix or staffing levels;
- changes in standards or outcome measures from local or national sources, e.g. national service frameworks.

Structure of ICP documentation

In general terms, ICP documents follow a defined structure which consists of:

- the front page(s) (patient details);
- clinical assessment (including risk assessment);
- patient management (including review points where the patient's progress is assessed allowing any remedial action to be taken);
- variations from the expected.

The front page(s) (patient details)

The front page(s) of an ICP document provides details about the patient, admission details and some background details about their condition and the intended management plan. Depending on the level of detail required, this section of the ICP might cover one or two pages. It should include (as appropriate to condition and care setting):

- patient details (name, address, home circumstances, past medical history, medication, allergies, next of kin, etc.);
- admission details (date, time and reason for admission);
- admission observations (temperature, pulse, etc.);
- diagnosis (for medical or community-based care) or intervention (for surgical or community-based care);
- desired objective of care;
- discharge criteria;
- expected length of stay;
- an appropriate statement regarding clinical judgement.

> An appropriate statement of clinical judgement:
>
> *'This pathway represents usual practice and variations are expected as clinicians use their own professional judgement.'*

This statement of clinical judgement is important as professional accountability is *increased* by the use of ICPs. At each stage of the pathway the responsible professional considers what is prescribed and asks, 'is this appropriate for the patient at this time?' If the answer is yes, then care continues as planned. If the

TOTAL HIP REPLACEMENT: PATHWAY
Desired Objective:

Unit No: Ward:	Consultant:
Surname:	Patient aware of planned care:
Forenames:	Hip booklet given: yes ❏
Address:	Date: / /
Telephone:	GP: Telephone:
Status: *M S W Other:*	Expected date of admission: / /
Age: Date of birth:	Expected date of discharge: / /
Religion:	
Occupation (past/present):	

HOME CIRCUMSTANCES/HOME ENVIRONMENT

Next of kin:

Relationship:
Address:

Telephone:
Alternative tel no:

Inform at night: Yes ❏   No ❏

Carer's health:

Other family dependents:

Problems caused by admission:

Relevant past medical history (brief details):

Family/carer understand reason for admission:

Yes ❏   No ❏

Family/carer understand planned care:

Yes ❏   No ❏

Accommodation: house/flat/bungalow/wc

Lives alone: Yes ❏   No ❏

Community care before admission

	Yes	No	Name (if poss)
Community nurse	❏	❏	
Home help	❏	❏	
Meals on wheels	❏	❏	
Social worker	❏	❏	
Health visitor	❏	❏	
CPN	❏	❏	

Information taken by	Grade:
Countersignature of trained nurse:	Date: / /

Figure 6.1 Sample front page

CLERKING OF MEDICAL HISTORY – UROLOGY

Presentation:

| **Previous history:** | **Surgical interventions:** |

Previous illness:

Asthma ❏	CVA ❏	HBP ❏	Epilepsy ❏
Angina ❏	COAD ❏	Rh.F ❏	Jaundice ❏
MI ❏	TB ❏	DU ❏	Diabetes ❏

Comments:

| **Family history:** | **Drug history:** |

| **Smoking history:**　y ❏　　n ❏ | **Alcohol history:**　y ❏　　n ❏ |

Systems review:

CVS:	RESP:
chest pain:	y ❏	n ❏	cough	y ❏	n ❏
dyspnoea:	y ❏	n ❏	sputum:	y ❏	n ❏
oedema:	y ❏	n ❏	wheezes:	y ❏	n ❏
Comments:			Comments:		

MEDICAL EXAMINATION

General examination:

Respiratory system:

CVS:
　Heart rate:　　　　　　　　　H/S:
　JVP:　　　　　　　　　　　　Oedema:

Abdomen:

CNS:

Figure 6.2 Sample medical assessment page

answer is no, the professional considers the alternative options and documents the course of action undertaken together with the reasons for the change(s).

A sample front page is shown in Figure 6.1.

Clinical assessment (including risk assessment)

Patient assessment tends to take place in three distinct stages:

- medical assessment
- nursing assessment
- therapy assessment.

In terms of an ICP, another stage of assessment can be identified:

- multidisciplinary assessment.

Medical assessment
Historically, medical assessment has been recorded on 'a blank piece of paper' and included in the medical case notes. Taking a medical history is a skill which doctors have learnt to complete using the systems in the human body. This provides for a full assessment, which, although it is thorough, may not be necessary or relevant for all patients or case types and may indeed be completed by nurses

who have received advanced training in assessment and diagnosis.

When an individual medical assessment is included in an ICP, details are entered onto a structured pro forma (Figure 6.2), agreed by senior medical staff and containing information relevant to the chosen client group. Time is saved by the use of a series of pre-defined questions and there is also less likelihood that something important will be missed.

Nursing assessment
Nursing assessment tends to follow activities of daily living in order to consider current activity and coping mechanisms prior to the onset of illness. These activities are usually defined as follows:

- breathing and circulation
- skin condition
- nutrition and fluids
- communication
- mobility
- elimination
- cognition
- sleep
- hygiene and dressing
- lifestyle
- social support.

NURSING ASSESSMENT: NUTRITION AND FLUIDS	
Usual condition	**On admission (within 12 hours)**
Special aid/help required yes ❏ no ❏	Special oral hygiene needs yes ❏ no ❏ specify: _____
Own teeth yes ❏ no ❏	Swallowing impaired yes ❏ no ❏
Dentures yes ❏ no ❏ good fit yes ❏ no ❏	(if yes completed speech and language referral today) referred yes ❏ no ❏
Mouthcare – independent yes ❏ no ❏	
Swallowing impaired yes ❏ no ❏	Nutritional risk score low ❏ medium ❏ high ❏
Special diet yes ❏ no ❏	Special diet yes ❏ no ❏
specify: _____	specify: _____
height _____	
weight _____	weight _____
Date Time	Signature

Figure 6.3 Nursing assessment (sample)

These activities can be built into the ICP to provide a basis for nursing assessment appropriate for the chosen client group (Figure 6.3).

Nursing assessment also incorporates risk assessment, using the following tools as required:

- nutritional assessment tool
- falls risk assessment tool
- pressure sore risk assessment tool
- pain assessment tool
- lifting and handling.

Therapy assessment
In general terms, therapy assessment focuses on functional ability (physiotherapy) and cognitive ability (occupational therapists) and the setting of appropriate goals for achievement. Therapists also usually keep their own, separately held, notes although they will often include information in the nursing notes if there is something specific they would like nurses to undertake or continue on their behalf. On some occasions nothing is written and the care provided by therapists is undertaken in isolation from the rest of the multidisciplinary team. Including this information in the ICP document, therefore, helps to integrate this care into the care cycle.

Multidisciplinary assessment
Undertaking separate medical, nursing and therapy assessments often results in duplication of information, with the patient answering the same question a number of different times. The use of ICPs offers the opportunity to introduce multidisciplinary assessment focusing on the presenting symptoms of the patient and the potential investigations and/or medication required. Responsibility for each assessment item can be indicated on the ICP (Dr, N, P, OT, SLT, etc. written next to each task) or a full assessment can be made by somebody trained to do so.

A sample multidisciplinary assessment page is shown in Figure 6.4.

Patient management
The patient management plan included in the ICP places the tasks, interventions and outcomes defined during 'getting started' against the expected time-frame for the pathway. More information on the time-frames used in ICPs can be found in the

section entitled *Sequential and appropriate care*, in **Chapter 1**.

There are a number of ways of presenting the management plan within the ICP. The example in Figure 6.5 specifies a management plan for each professional group involved in providing care. When management plans are presented in this way they are often colour coded by professional to simplify access to the relevant information.

Alternatively, another common method entails specifying the management plan by 'aspects of care' (Figure 6.6).

For more complex and less predictable patient groups it may be appropriate to consider patient needs and activities of daily living together with more traditional clinical management plans (Figure 6.7). Their use will help to measure the progress of the patient along the pathway.

In addition to recording tasks, interventions and outcomes, the patient management plans should include space for each professional group to record additional comments (often called *progress notes* or *communication*) as appropriate. If the patient is progressing as planned there is no need to write any progress notes. This space is generally used to communicate information to other professionals (e.g. a message) or to highlight any issues raised by the patient or their family. The recording of additional comments should be based on 'exception reporting', a discipline many professionals find difficult to follow during the first few weeks of using a pathway. The temptation exists to record the relevant information within the patient management plan and to *also* summarize this within the progress notes. Exception reporting becomes easier with time once each professional begins to feel confident that nothing pertinent is being missed.

Progress notes are generally presented opposite the patient management plans and there are two main ways of recording this information. Firstly, progress notes can be 'split' by professional group (Figure 6.8).

More commonly, progress notes are recorded on a multidisciplinary progress sheet (Figure 6.9).

Figure 6.10 presents sample ICP pages for assessment, management and discharge.

Variations from the expected

Recording variations from the expected patient management plan is essential to the

---

PRE-OPERATIVE PATIENT ASSESSMENT

NAME: WARD:

Breathing: Smoker ❑   Non-smoker ❑   **Allergies:**
Breathless on exertion: Yes ❑   No ❑
Cough   Yes ❑   No ❑
Predisposing chest condition: (see Pharmacy Sheet)

Mouth (any problems with mouth/teeth/dentures?)
Caries   ❑   Own teeth   ❑
Crowns   ❑   Dentures   ❑ with patient   yes ❑   no ❑

Communicate and interact with others:

Sight:	**Hearing:** Good ❑ Poor ❑
Registered blind ❑	Aids used: Yes ❑ No ❑
Partially sighted ❑	
Good vision ❑	**Speech** Clear: Yes ❑ No ❑
	Deficit:
Wears glasses: ❑	
Reading ❑	**Mental state**
Constant ❑	Sensible ❑
with patient yes ❑ no ❑	Uncooperative ❑
Wears contact lenses: ❑	Mildly confused ❑
with patient yes ❑ no ❑	Aggressive ❑
	Confused ❑

Eating and drinking:
Appetite: Good ❑   Poor ❑
Type of diet (specify):
Supplementary foods needed: Yes ❑   No ❑   Refer to dietician: ❑
Help needed with feeding: Yes ❑   No ❑
Special equipment used (specify):

Elimination:

Bladder:		**Bowels:**	
Normal	❑	Normal	❑
Incontinent	❑	Loose stool	❑
Catheter	❑	Constipation	❑
Ileostomy	❑	Colostomy	❑
Nocturia	❑	Other:	

Mobility

Limp	❑	Stairs:		Bed bound ❑
No aids	❑	No problem	❑	
One stick	❑	Some	❑	
Two sticks	❑	Difficult	❑	
Crutches	❑	Impossible	❑	
Wheelchair	❑			
Frame	❑			

Sleeping:

Well	❑		Sleeps in:	
On medication	❑	Please specify: (on Pharmacy sheet)	Bed	❑
Interrupted sleep	❑		Chair:	❑
Does not sleep	❑		Other:	❑

Information taken by   Grade:

Countersignature of trained nurse: Date: /   /

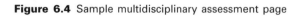

Figure 6.4 Sample multidisciplinary assessment page

FRACTURED NECK OF FEMUR - Postoperative day 3
Medical Management 1. [*intervention*] 2. [*intervention*] 3. [*outcome*]
Nursing Management 1. [*intervention*] 2. [*intervention*] 3. [*outcome*]
Physiotherapy Management 1. [*intervention*] 2. [*intervention*] 3. [*outcome*]
Occupational Therapy Management 1. [*intervention*] 2. [*intervention*] 3. [*outcome*]
Comments

Figure 6.5 Sample management plan (by professional group)

SURGERY	Postoperative day 2	Signature
Assessment	[*intervention*] [*outcome*]	
Investigation(s)	[*intervention*] [*outcome*]	
Treatment	[*intervention*] [*outcome*]	
Drugs	[*intervention*] [*outcome*]	
Mobility	[*intervention*] [*outcome*]	
Diet	[*intervention*] [*outcome*]	
Teaching/psychological support	[*intervention*] [*outcome*]	
Discharge planning	[*intervention*] [*outcome*]	

Figure 6.6 Sample management plan (by aspects of care)

STROKE – Day 2	
Assessment • [*intervention*]	outcome:
Communication • [*intervention*]	outcome:
Medication • [*intervention*]	outcome:
Nutrition • [*intervention*]	outcome:
Mobility • [*intervention*]	outcome:
Elimination • [*intervention*]	outcome:
Personal hygiene • [*intervention*]	outcome:
Psychological care • [*intervention*]	outcome:
Social care/discharge planning • [*intervention*]	outcome:
Communication with family • [*intervention*]	outcome:

Figure 6.7 Sample management plan (more complex patient groups)

PROGRESS NOTES – Day 3
MEDICAL REVIEW signature and time
NURSING REVIEW signature and time
PHYSIOTHERAPY REVIEW signature and time
OCCUPATIONAL THERAPY REVIEW signature and time
OTHER signature and time

Figure 6.8 Progress notes split by professional group

Date and time	Multidisciplinary progress notes – **Day 2**	Signature and profession

Figure 6.9 Progress notes recorded on a multidisciplinary progress sheet

successful use of ICPs. In keeping with the options available for presenting patient management plans, there are a number of ways variations from the expected can be recorded in the ICP document. For example, a section for variations can be added to the multidisciplinary progress sheet (Figure 6.11).

The advantage of this approach is that variations are recorded daily at the time they occur. The disadvantage, however, is that once the page is turned, other members of staff may not be aware that a variation has occurred.

A second option is to record variations on the same page as the patient management plan (Figure 6.12).

Whichever option is used to record variations from the expected, it is usual to include a separate page to record variations at the back of the ICP document (Figure 6.13). Here the variations can be re-written and coded as appropriate to support ICP reviews and audit.

The coding of variations (see figure 6.14) helps the multi-disciplinary team to identify trends, which may be resolved by amending the pathway or the interventions included in the patient management plan. Care must be taken when recording variations, particularly in a busy clinical area, to avoid problems with the accuracy of data.

In terms of defining codes to represent variations from the expected, there are two main issues to resolve at a local level, namely:

- *How many codes to use?* A small number of codes makes for both simpler data collection and input. However, the possibility exists that using too few codes restricts the ability to accurately record variations and to identify any meaningful trends on analysis. Conversely, using too many codes can be time consuming and also increases the chances of the wrong codes being used. A balance needs to be established according to local conditions with the aim being to use the minimum number of codes to comprehensively and accurately record any variations that occur.
- *Who is responsible for coding?* There are a number of options to consider when deciding who is responsible for coding:
  - the clinician who identifies the variation
  - the nurse manager codes on a daily basis
  - clinical nurse specialists code on daily basis
  - audit staff code from a brief description provided by staff.

It is often simpler if variations are recorded by the responsible clinician and are translated into codes by a member of staff trained to carry out this task. It is worth remembering, however, that the more ICPs are used, the more variations will need to be coded and this option may equate to the appointment of a specific member of staff to be responsible for coding. Again, local circumstances need to be taken into consideration (case mix, experience of staff, number of ICPs in use, resources available) in order to resolve this issue in the safest and most reliable manner.

Generalizability of ICP documentation

Whilst the content of different ICPs will obviously differ according to clinical

Paediatric Asthma Care Pathway

Unit number:
Name:
Address:

Date of birth:

Label

Date: [   ]   Booking time: [   ]

Time seen by triage nurse: [   ]

Nurse code: [   ]

Patient accompanied by:

Nurse Assessment – If a box marked [Y] is ticked, the patient must be seen by a doctor immediately
This may be LIFE THREATENING.

Known asthma patient	N [ ]	Y [ ]

1. Colour:	Cyanosed:	N [ ]	* Y [ ]

2. Physical state:	Normal	Y [ ]	N [ ]
	Breathless	N [ ]	Y [ ]
	Agitated or reduced conscious level	N [ ]	* Y [ ]
	Exhausted or fatigued	N [ ]	* Y [ ]

3. Ability to speak/babble	Normal	Y [ ]	N [ ]
	With difficulty/unable	N [ ]	Y [ ]

4. Ability to walk/feed:	Normal	Y [ ]	N [ ]
	With difficulty/unable	N [ ]	Y [ ]

5. Observations:	Using accessory muscles:		N [ ]	Y [ ]
	Respiration rate: [ ]	Below 50	Y [ ]	N [ ]
	Heart rate: [ ]	Below 140	Y [ ]	N [ ]
	Temperature: [ ]			

6. Peak flow measurement: (over 5 years of age)

Previously used peak flow meter? Y [ ]   N [ ]

Able to do peak flow? Y [ ]   N [ ]

Predicted/best: [   ]   Actual: [   ]

Above 50% predicted Y [ ]   N [ ]
Above 33% predicted Y [ ]   * N [ ]

---

7. Oxygen saturation: [   ] %   Above 92% Y [ ]   N [ ]

Oxygen saturation measured in air Y [ ]   or specify oxygen given: [   ]

Give oxygen via face mask to maintain above 92% and specify oxygen given: [   ]

---

8. Classification

Mild [ ]	Moderate/severe [ ]	Life threatening * [ ]
See doctor: **Within 1 hour**	**Within 10 mins**	**IMMEDIATELY**

---

9. Time of referral to doctor: [   ]   Time of referral to paeds if life threatening: [   ]

Figure 6.10 Sample ICP – assessment, management and discharge

Medical Assessment

| Seen by: *print name* | | Time: | |

History

Symptoms during this attack

	Cough		Wheeze		Breathless
Day		Day		Day	
Night		Night		Night	
Exercise		Exercise		Exercise	

Night time wakening due to:

Cough [ ] Wheeze [ ] Breathless [ ]

Duration of this attack:

Days [ ] Hours [ ]

In the last six months:

No. of emergency visits GP [ ] Hospital [ ] No. of admissions to hospital: [ ]

Has the child ever been admitted to ITU with asthma? Yes [ ] No [ ]

Regular treatment:	Drug	Device/route	Dose	Frequency
Reliever:				
Preventer:				

Treatment in this attack: no. of doses in last 24 hours

Reliever:				
Preventer:				
Prednisolone:				

Examination:

Colour:	Cyanosed	N [ ]	* Y [ ]
Physical state:	Normal	Y [ ]	N [ ]
	Breathless	N [ ]	Y [ ]
	Agitated/reduced conscious level	N [ ]	* Y [ ]
	Exhausted/fatigued	N [ ]	* Y [ ]
Ability to speak/babble:	Normal	Y [ ]	N [ ]
	With difficulty/unable	N [ ]	Y [ ]
Respiration:	Using accessory muscles	N [ ]	Y [ ]

Figure 6.10 (*continued*) Sample ICP – assessment, management and discharge

Other: *record observations in column below

Diagnosis: | **Sign:** | | **Time:** |

Management

Prednisolone: Dose: Sign: If not given, reason:

Time given: Sign:

Nebulizer before hospital	**First nebulizer**	**Second nebulizer**
N ☐ Y ☐	Drug:	Dose:
	Dose: Sign:	Dose: Sign:
Time given: ☐	Time given: ☐ Sign:	Time given: ☐ Sign:

Observations on examination	**Discharge criteria**	**After 1st nebulizer**	**Discharge criteria**	**After 2nd nebulizer**	**Discharge criteria**
Time: ☐		Time: ☐		Time: ☐	
Peak flow: ☐	above 50% ☐	☐	above 50% ☐	☐	above 50% ☐
SaO$_2$ (in air) ☐	above 92% ☐	☐	above 92% ☐	☐	above 92% ☐
Resp. rate ☐	below 50/min ☐	☐	below 50/min ☐	☐	below 50/min ☐
Pulse rate: ☐	below 140/min ☐	☐	below 140/min ☐	☐	below 140/min ☐
Absence of asthma symptoms (See 2, 3, 4 page 1) ☐		Absence of asthma symptoms (See 2, 3, 4 page 1) ☐		Absence of asthma symptoms (See 2, 3, 4 page 1) ☐	

Action:

Discharge: ☐
(all discharge criteria met)

Nebulize: ☐
(mild/mod/severe)

Refer to paeds: ☐
(mod/severe)

Discharge: ☐
(all discharge criteria met)

Nebulize: ☐
(mild/mod/severe)

Refer to paeds: ☐
(mod/severe)

Discharge: ☐
(all discharge criteria met)

Nebulize: ☐
(mild/mod/severe)

Paeds/med assessment   Time referred to paediatrician: ☐

Action: Admit: ☐   Discharge: ☐   – complete discharge criteria

| **Name:** | **Sign:** | **Time:** |

Figure 6.10 (*continued*) Sample ICP – assessment, management and discharge

	Discharge			
Treatment for discharge				
	Drug	**Strength/dose**	**Route/device**	**Frequency**
Reliever				
Preventer				
Prednisolone				
Other				

Checklist

Prednisolone prescribed ☐

Bronchodilator prescribed ☐

Asthma education

      treatment explanation ☐

      advice sheet given ☐

      inhaler technique checked ☐

Self management plan ☐

GP letter ☐

Follow-up

See GP ☐

Refer to respiratory team ☐

OPD – Paediatricians only ☐

Time of discharge ☐

Print name/ designation ☐

Signature: ☐

Comments

Figure 6.10 (*continued*) Sample ICP – assessment, management and discharge

Date and time	Multidisciplinary progress notes – Day 2		Signature and profession
	Variations from expected management plan	**Action taken**	

Figure 6.11 Recording variations on the multidisciplinary progress sheet

STROKE – Day 2		Variations
Assessment • [*intervention*]	outcome:	
Communication • [*intervention*]	outcome:	
Medication • [*intervention*]	outcome:	
Nutrition • [*intervention*]	outcome:	
Mobility • [*intervention*]	outcome:	
Elimination • [*intervention*]	outcome:	
Personal hygiene • [*intervention*]	outcome:	
Psychological care • [*intervention*]	outcome:	
Social care/discharge planning • [*intervention*]	outcome:	
Communication with family • [*intervention*]	outcome:	

Figure 6.12 Recording variations with the patient management plan

Date	Variation	Code	Cause	Action taken	Resolution	Signature Profession

Figure 6.13 Sample variations page (to include at the back of ICP document)

Clinical condition
1. DVT suspected
2. High Temperature
3.
4.
5. Patient mobilized earlier than expected
6.

Patient/family/carer
7.
8. Inadequate carer support
9. Patient refused treatment
10.
11.

Clinician
12. No physiotherapist available
13.
14.
15.

Systems
16.
17. Inadequate information
18.
19.

External systems
20.
21. Inadequate access to home
22.
23.

Figure 6.14 Sample codes for variations from the expected

condition/client group, it is helpful for organizations to consider developing a standard format for all ICPs in use at a particular location. Familiarity with the documentation can help to ease difficult situations and safeguard patients when:

- patients are placed into a different specialty from the one into which they were admitted
- staff rotation takes place between specialties
- staff shortages occur or there is a high number of bank staff.

A number of organizations have found it helpful to colour code the different sections included within ICP documentation, for example, as follows:

- the front page(s)   = yellow pages
  (patient details)
- clinical and nursing   = green pages
  assessment
- patient management   = pink pages
- variations from the   = blue pages.
  expected

Patient information – the development of patient pathways

Introduction

In terms of providing information to patients about their condition and expected treatment, the use of patient pathways is an important option to consider. Patient pathways are presented in the same format as an ICP and are intended to replace more traditional forms of patient information, with its content to be discussed with the patient at the earliest available opportunity.

The patient is encouraged to complete their pathway as an integral part of their care, building into a 'diary of events'. This information can be shared with staff on a day-to-day basis to ensure there are no misunderstandings and that the patient understands what is happening, when, where and by whom. In addition, the patient pathway can be collected on discharge as part of an audit of patient perspectives. The pathway can also move with the patient around the health arena to support the process of multidisciplinary and multi-agency collaboration.

Writing a patient pathway

A patient pathway should include:

- an introduction to patient pathways
- guidance for using the patient pathway
- a description of the nature of ICPs and their use
- details on where the ICP will be kept
- information on the patient's condition and their treatment
- information to describe variations from the expected and how care is individualized to suit patient needs.

An introduction to patient pathways

> The staff who are looking after you whilst you are in hospital have put together this patient pathway to help you understand what is happening to you during your stay with us.

Guidance for using the patient pathway

> Your patient pathway is there for you to read and complete. Please think of it as a diary of events and use it to write down any impressions you have about your care. You may choose to use the blank space to write down any questions that you wish to ask the staff. You may wish to tell us what you thought of your care – good and bad. If there is something we could have done better or differently we would be pleased to hear about it.
>
> It would also be really useful if your comments were discussed with the staff who are caring for you. Do not worry if you feel that you are criticizing us – if we do not get feedback on our care we cannot change those things that require changing.

A description of the nature of ICPs and their use

> An ICP is a plan of care which has been written by doctors, nurses, therapists and other professionals involved in your treatment. It lists the tasks to be performed at specified times of your stay and the outcomes you can expect to achieve to help you through your stay in hospital. It is used by staff to record your care at each stage of your stay and is the legal record of the care you receive during your stay with us.

Details on where the ICP will be kept

> The ICP is kept at your bedside. Please read it. The nurses and doctors will be happy to explain any part of the ICP to you or answer any questions you may have.
>
> **NB If the ICP is kept away from the patient, you may wish to explain why this is so**

Information on the patient's condition and their treatment
An example is shown in Figure 6.15.

On the day of your admission to the ward	Please tick everything that has been carried out. Write any comments or questions you may have in the space below
the ward staff will: • show you around the ward • introduce you to other patients • measure and record your blood pressure, pulse and temperature • answer any questions you may have in relation to your stay in hospital and your discharge from hospital • expected discharge date:	
your surgeon will: • explain your operation to you and ask you sign a form to say that you understand and agree to the operation • answer any questions you may have in relation to your operation	
your anaesthetist will: • ensure that you are fit for anaesthetic • answer any questions that you may have in relation to the anaesthetic	
In preparation for theatre you will: • wear a wristband which includes your name, date of birth and hospital number • shave your skin around your operation site • eat nothing from _____ am/pm • be given a sleeping tablet to help you sleep (optional)	
Outcome of the day: _____will have been seen by ward staff, doctor and anaesthetist and understands his/her operation	**Outcomes met:** yes ❏　　　　　no ❏

Figure 6.15 Patient pathway example: surgical procedure requiring a general anaesthetic

Information to describe variations from the expected and how care is individualized to suit patient needs

You are a unique person to us and so is everyone that comes into the hospital and we will always treat you as an individual. However, in relation to the reason for your hospital treatment, we know that there are certain investigations, medication and procedures that you must receive during your stay. These are recorded in your ICP. Not all patients will follow the ICP exactly, and if there need to be any changes to the treatment plan we will explain why this has happened and what action we are taking. This does not necessarily mean that there is something wrong or that you will not be able to go home as arranged. If you have any questions or concerns about your ICP or changes in treatment please do discuss this with us.

Patient information guidelines

In keeping with other forms of patient information, patient pathways should be written using the following guidelines (Henderson, 1999):

- Use direct language addressing the reader as 'you' or 'your' and not 'the patient/s'.
- Avoid language that may cause offence, e.g. 'a person who has epilepsy' and not 'the epileptic'.
- Avoid unnecessary abbreviations, e.g. 'Special Care Baby Unit' not 'SCBU'.
- Present risks and areas of scientific uncertainty as numbers not percentages, e.g. '18 out of 20' not '90 per cent'.
- Explain medical terminology and do not use medical jargon.
- Use everyday words and avoid unfamiliar ones.
- Use active verbs.
- Avoid unnecessary fillers.

Conclusions

This chapter has shown that there are many ways of presenting ICP documentation. The key to success is local determination of the issues involved as it is at a local level these documents will be in day-to-day use. In essence, the documentation must be accepted and 'owned' by the clinical staff involved. However, it is important to remember that, as a minimum, ICP documentation *should* be:

- user-friendly
- sequential
- outcome-based
- evidence-based
- flexible
- easily audited, and
- transferable to other clinical areas within the same organization.

Reference

Henderson, Diane, Jones, Julie, and Lord, Sue (1999) *'Don't let the ink dry': guidelines for the production of good quality condition-specific patient information.* Wrexham, North East Wales NHS Trust.

7

Crossing professional and service boundaries: a case study

Leslie Braidwood and Tracy P. Evans

Introduction

In this chapter we present our strategy and experience of setting up integrated care pathways (ICPs) within the health care community in Doncaster. We will present an overview of our stance, a summary list of features relating to ICPs and other organizational systems we have introduced, showing their benefits, and finally outline a practical example of ICP generation in a clinical setting.

Background and general viewpoint (the strategy)

In Doncaster we are uniquely placed to explore and develop seamless primary, intermediate and secondary care. In the Acute Trust we have had established pathways for chronic diseases for three years. In the past two years we have also had a primary care-based initiative – APPROACH (Agreed Pathways and PROtocols for Accessing Care in Health) – which has addressed the problems of increasing waiting lists by a pathway-based multi-professional net of service delivery points. Our most recent innovation is to begin the joining of APPROACH pathways with existing and yet-to-be-developed secondary care ICPs to provide optimum use of resources, and measurable systems for quality management, which are based on outcome rather than activity.

We have developed joint working teams, which are all multi-boundary and multi-professional. Each is led by one individually picked 'eager champion' and covers a limited area of disease management, e.g., cardio-vascular disease, in which there is the simultaneous development of guidelines, referral patterns and in-hospital pathways. This allows for uniform patient handling with appropriate and effective service provision by doctor-led and non-doctor-led teams. The 'champion' provides the driving force and energy, ensuring that the momentum of change is maintained; the team structure ensures that no professional viewpoint is overlooked, and the multi-boundary involvement decreases time and work wastage by ensuring appropriate care. A structured mix of whole-group and sub-group activities ensures the continuity of development so that within any single-disease care process a proper balance is maintained between detail and strategy.

In developing these structures we have met gratifyingly little tribalism and less inertia because we have deliberately designed teams to deliver 'all-stakeholder-benefit' outcomes where no individual or group is allowed to be a loser. We have paced change at an optimum but not maximal rate and have thus kept leading- and trailing-edge participants comfortable with progress as it is made. Problems have arisen, as would be expected when expensive capital investments are needed, and we have had to deliberately win over some authority figures who are not directly involved in the process and therefore view it as innovative and suspicious. But, on the whole, we have encountered much less resistance because we consistently *headline* our objectives to all participants and ensure that our objectives are deliverable, so that everyone in a team knows what they are supposed to be doing and where they are going.

As a result of this open attitude, gains have been made by all users. Patients are seen more quickly while consultants now see patients who are more appropriate to their skill level.

Nursing staff and PAMs (professions allied to medicine) have seen a development in their role and empowerment. General practitioners (GPs) have found multiple structures available for the care of their patients so that they become route-planners not gatekeepers; lastly, managers and their support staff have found structures and design where before there was a morass.

Summary listing of ICP features

Why use ICPs and why develop APPROACH?

- Delivers all the benefits of pathways of care.
- Makes interface problems a thing of the past by developing continuous care.
- Allows quality management to develop in a measurable environment.

How do we develop them?

- Contact interested people across every boundary and select a core team of motivated people who can motivate others.
- Choose clinical areas where you are very likely to succeed (delivered success promotes future success).
- Have a strategy group which is practical.
- Set a workable timetable and keep to it (limit your ambitions to what you can achieve).

Problems and delights

Delights
- Always spread good news.
- Develop teams and encourage sharing.
- Never isolate a person, department or service.

Problems
- Have the strategy group list all problems and all risks (people, procedures, inertia, cost, etc.).
- Have practical fall-back positions so that every attempted project can be completed (don't climb insurmountable rock faces!).
- When problems occur deal with them quickly, and make common solutions so that everyone benefits and feels better.

The benefits of the process

For NHS personnel
- More effective working.
- An enhanced sense of achievement (more deliverables).
- Belonging to a team.
- Greatly diminished 'conflict' in the workplace.

For NHS management
- Systems that managers can understand.
- A change from process measurement to outcome measurement.
- A more self-reliant workforce.
- Possibility of developing staff.

For the patient
- Easier access to care and speedier care.
- Care which is more understandable.
- Usually, if working well, a friendlier atmosphere.

Setting up an ICP in a defined clinical setting

We feel that it is important to only develop ICPs which are relevant to clinical practice and which will show direct measurable benefit to all stakeholders. An analysis of our clinical indicators within the Acute Trust showed an unexpectedly high incidence of grommet insertion in children with otitis media with effusion (OME). Preliminary discussions with each of the consultants in the Ear, Nose and Throat Department (ENT) emphasized their opinion that the operating frequency was based on sound clinical practice and that the excess in service delivery reflected excess need and demand for treatment by patients. At the instigation of one of the consultant ENT surgeons an audit of sweep hearing tests in children of school entry age was completed, the results of which are shown in Figure 7.1.

Of the 104 children seen by a GP and referred to the ENT department, 38 per cent (40 children) required surgery.

The recommendations of the audit were for the adherence to a systematic approach when dealing with OME. Protocols existed for in-hospital treatment and the assessment of children within the school nursing service; no protocol existed for the handling of OME in

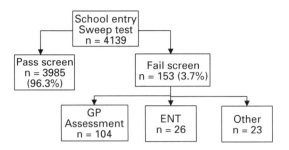

Figure 7.1 School entry sweep test results

primary care. This meant equity of access could not be ensured for all patients reaching our ENT service and parts of the services possessed tighter measures of quality assurance than others. In one of those serendipitous events which begin projects, one of the consultant ENT team decided to establish an ICP for the treatment of OME. This would extend from any patient presentation through primary care and secondary care to provide an auditable, secure and equitable service pathway for all the patients.

An initial consultative group, which developed into the steering committee for the ICP, was formed from all ENT consultants, ICP co-ordinator, GPs, chief and paediatric audiologists, paediatric nurses, and representatives from theatre, recovery and anaesthetics. As work progressed, the steering committee co-opted representatives from the School Nurse Service and Nurse Management from the Healthcare Trust.

The steering group resolved that the following should be the backbone of the ICP:

1 The patient record should be reconstructed to provide a chronological record of their illness and management with the absolute minimum of duplication of clinical information. This implied a change in the sense of ownership of medical, nursing and PAM records, which explicitly demonstrated the closeness of team working within the single OME ICP. This process involved much discussion, some horse-trading, and eventually the agreed loss of some cherished areas of ownership. It was encouraging but not surprising that consequently all members of the steering group accepted the principle of a commonly held chronological single case note.

2 A rigid flow diagram demonstrating the movement of patients from any entry point through the management process of the ICP was developed.

3 All significant events or care processes within the ICP should be measurable. An audit structure, which defines standards of quality of performance, should be attached to these events and processes.

4 A practicable and workable timetable for the implementation of the ICP was agreed.

5 For all new procedures or revisions of existing procedures appropriate in-service training was provided, this was particularly important for secondary care nursing staff as the final clinical documentation which we use differs in a number of respects from the nursing process of which they were familiar. A number of GPs who provide in-service audiometry were given advice on the difficulties and limitations of this procedure to ensure that no excessively high expectation of quality was placed on these measurements, which are almost always uncertainly controlled.

6 Marketing the ICP was actively discussed in the steering group and a number of multi-boundary difficulties were discovered which could not be resolved. It was comparatively easy to highlight the ICP within secondary care and each professional discipline took over the responsibility of within-department marketing. A major problem remained with marketing the ICP to first-degree care, for at the time of development TARGET (Time for Audit, Review, Guidelines, Education and Training), which is now our main inter-boundary change organ, had not yet been formed. It was suggested that an approved referral letter be designed and circulated to GPs as an interim measure.

Following the initial work of the steering group, small sub-committees were set up, each drawing its membership partly from the steering group and co-opted additional professionals, as necessary, to deal with specific departmental and sub-departmental issues. This proved extremely valuable in developing a sense of belonging to a team and in preparing the common clinical record. Without too much slippage, draft and revisions were prepared, reviewed and combined to form the paper-base for the ICP.

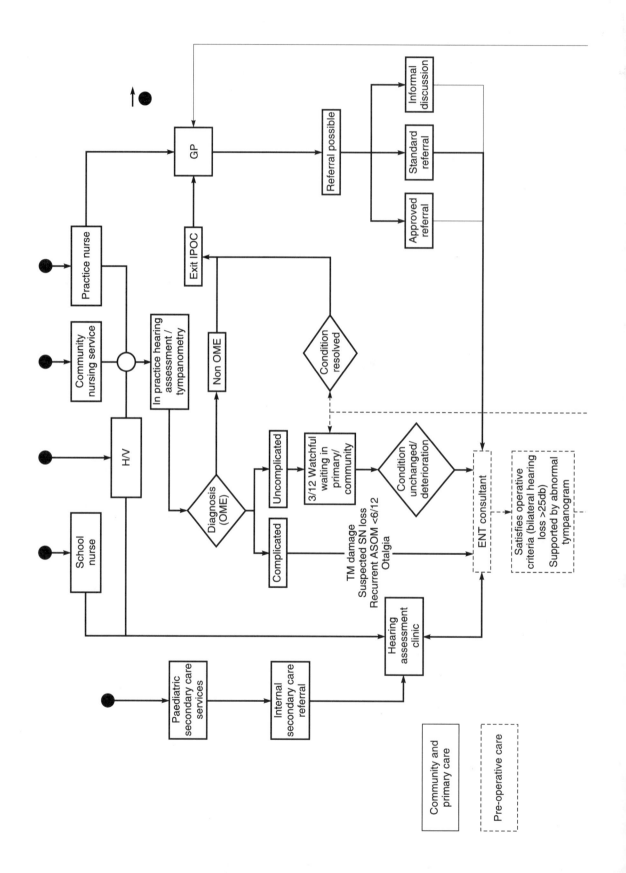

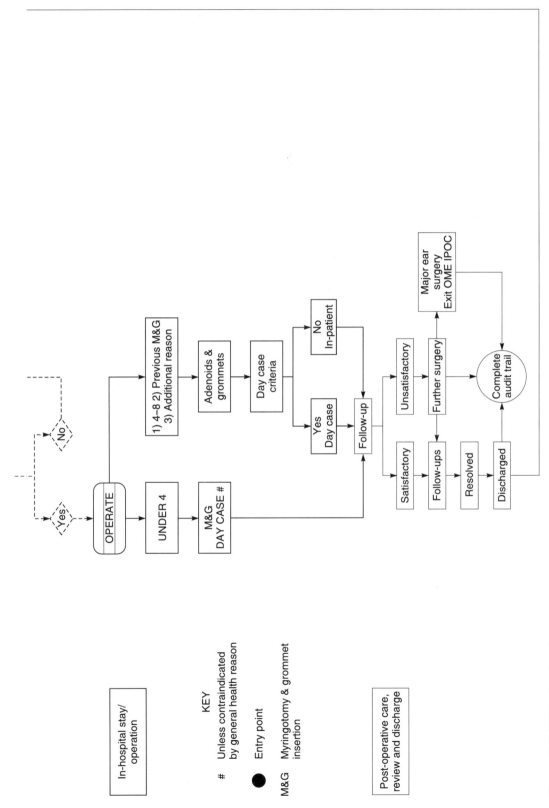

Figure 7.2 OME referral pathway

At the end of this process one persistent problem remained in the fact that the anaesthetic department required a one-page anaesthetic sheet rather than the customary large anaesthetic document and this could not be fitted chronologically in the ICP and meet the storage requirements of the records department. It is therefore detached from the ICP and stored separately in the medical notes.

Outcomes

The OME ICP has not been in place sufficiently long to produce statistical evidence in the change of care provision. However, preliminary review of the data in accordance with the measurables and auditables decided upon by the steering group points to a 20 per cent (ball-park) reduction in grommet insertion without any change in re-referrals for management of 'not-yet-resolved' problems. This represents an exciting and satisfactory outcome from the ICP as it demonstrates that, even when carefully appraised by competent experts' opinions, relating to 'how we do it around here' can be wrong. (None of the medical, nursing and support teams felt there was an

excess of grommet insertion, rationalizing that they simply did more because there were more to do.) However, our preliminary data suggests that grommet insertions have declined without loss of clinical quality or increases in alternative treatments.

The team has implemented a flexible and adaptable change in standard setting and clinical behaviour, which (according to our preliminary indications) will deliver improved service and better quality assessment for OME patients.

Conclusions

The setting up of ICPs provides the most appropriate tool for changing the process of care provision. It allows change to occur within safe and structured confines, without exposing patients to risk and without threatening employees (in whatever discipline) with excessive or unachievable challenges.

The example we provide demonstrates the central role for a 'champion' who drives the process for the development of a team consisting of all stakeholders – and ensures the setting of timed deliverables which are within the scope of the team as a whole.

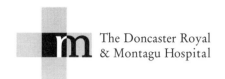
The Doncaster Royal
& Montagu Hospital

Pilot Document

Otitis Media with Effusion

*Integrated Pathway of Care
for children (0 - 16 years)*

**If you have any problems,
please contact Tracy Evans Ext. 3820**

Figure 7.3 ICP pilot document: otitis media with effusion

The Doncaster Royal & Montagu Hospital

CONTENTS

AFFIX LABEL HERE IF AVAILABLE

Unit Number...

Surname...

Forename(s)..

HMR

Page	Completed	N/A	Title
1.	☐	☐	Hearing Concern Sheet
2.	☐	☐	ENT History
3.	☐	☐	Hearing Assessment - Pure Tone
4.	☐	☐	Hearing Assessment - Distraction Test
5.	☐	☐	Deafness Concern
6.	☐	☐	Medical Examination
7.	☐	☐	Admission of ENT Patients
8.	☐	☐	Physical Examination
9.	☐	☐	ENT Assessment
10.	☐	☐	Admission
11.	☐	☐	ADL Assessment
12.	☐	☐	Admission Day
13.	☐	☐	Theatre
14.	☐	☐	Return to Ward
15.	☐	☐	Continuation Notes
16.	☐	☐	Discharge
17.	☐	☐	Hearing Assessment - Pure Tone
18.	☐	☐	Hearing Assessment - Distraction Test
19.	☐	☐	Audit Trail

Return to IPOC Co-ordinator

Figure 7.3 (*continued*)

The Doncaster Royal
& Montagu Hospital

HEARING CONCERN SHEET

Unit Number..

Surname..

Forename(s)..

Date of initial visit: .... Referred by: .... Designation:...................

G.P.: ....

Reason: ....

....

Siblings:

Family History of hearing loss ?   No ☐   Yes ☐   ....

Birth History: Date of Birth: ....

Birth weight: ....   Maturity:.............................   weeks

Insignificant NNU ☐

Significant NNU ☐   Ventilation ☐

Exchange transfusion ☐

Significant infection ☐

Other ☐

Pregnancy Illnesses: Pre-natal infection ☐

Diabetes ☐

Rubella ☐   Rubella contact ☐

Mother immunised ☐

Previous History: Ear infections ☐   Mumps ☐

Respiratory infections ☐   Measles ☐

Urinary infections ☐   Meningitis ☐

Fits ☐

Significant conditions: ....

Developmental milestones (see Protocol):

Speech and language milestones

Babble ☐   Meaningful words: ....

Two words together ☐   Small Sentences ☐   Full sentences ☐

Understanding of language: age-appropriate ?   Yes ☐   No ☐

Parents' opinion regarding hearing:

Referred to ENT
Consultant ?
Yes / No

Cons: ....

Date: ....

History of recent illness:

Page 1.   Signature: ....   Print Name: ....

Figure 7.3 (*continued*)

	AFFIX LABEL HERE IF AVAILABLE	HMR
m The Doncaster Royal & Montagu Hospital	Unit Number..	
	Surname...	
ENT HISTORY	Forename(s)...	

New Patient Questionnaire returned ?   Yes / No   If yes, attach to sheet

Previously seen by ENT Surgeon ?   Yes / No   If yes, please give details below

Date		Signature

Page 2.

Figure 7.3 (*continued*)

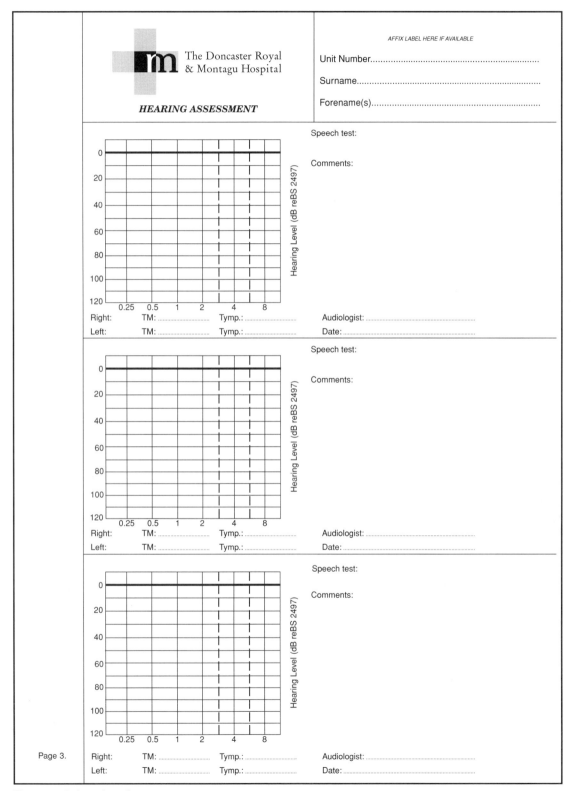

Figure 7.3 (*continued*)

The Doncaster Royal
& Montagu Hospital

HEARING ASSESSMENT

Unit Number...

Surname..

Forename(s)...

Comments:

Right Binaural Left

Warble 0.5KHz

Warble 2.0KHz

Warble 4.0KHz

High-frequency rattle

Location

Speech test

Right: TM: ....   Tymp.: ....   Audiologist: ....

Left: TM: ....   Tymp.: ....   Date: ....

Comments:

Right Binaural Left

Warble 0.5KHz

Warble 2.0KHz

Warble 4.0KHz

High-frequency rattle

Location

Speech test

Right: TM: ....   Tymp.: ....   Audiologist: ....

Left: TM: ....   Tymp.: ....   Date: ....

Comments:

Right Binaural Left

Warble 0.5KHz

Warble 2.0KHz

Warble 4.0KHz

High-frequency rattle

Location

Speech test

Right: TM: ....   Tymp.: ....   Audiologist: ....

Left: TM: ....   Tymp.: ....   Date: ....

Page 4.

Figure 7.3 (*continued*)

The Doncaster Royal
& Montagu Hospital

DEAFNESS CONCERN

AFFIX LABEL HERE IF AVAILABLE

Unit Number..

Surname...

Forename(s)..

Source of referral:

CMO ☐   GP ☐   Other: ....   Family History ?   Yes / No

....

Duration suspected   < 6 months ☐   Fluctuant ☐   Persistent ☐

                               > 6 months ☐

Side: Right / Left / Both / Don't know

Associated effects:		**Associated symptoms:**	
Speech delay	☐	Otitis Media	☐
Educational delay	☐	Nasal Obstruction	☐
Behavioural disorder	☐	Snores	☐
		Rhinorrhoea	
		Tonsilitis	☐
		Asthma	☐

Past Medical History:

		reatment:
Measles	☐	
Mumps	☐	
Meningitis	☐	
Head Trauma	☐	
Other:	☐	

Previous hearing tests ?   Yes / No   7 month screen   Pass / Fail

....

Others:

Previous T	**No**	**Yes**	**Date**
Grommets	☐	☐	....
Adenoidectomy	☐	☐	....
Tonsillectomy	☐	☐	....

Page 5.

Figure 7.3 (*continued*)

The Doncaster Royal & Montagu Hospital

MEDICAL EXAMINATION

AFFIX LABEL HERE IF AVAILABLE

Unit Number...

Surname...

Forename(s)..

Date: ....

Tympanic membrane:

Perforated ?   Yes / No

Atelectasis ?   Yes / No

SADE Grade: ....

TOS Grade: ....

RIGHT   **LEFT**

For definition
see Protocol

SADE I
         II
         III
         IV

TOS   I
         II
         III

Syndrome: Cleft ☐   Downs ☐   Other: ....

(Suspected i.e. dysmorphism)

Nasal Airway: Normal ☐   Restricted ☐

Palate: Normal ☐
                 Abnormal ☐   Submucous cleft ☐
                                  Bifid Uvula ☐
                                  Repaired cleft ☐

Hearing test: Normal ☐
                       Abnormal ☐

Compliance: A ☐   B ☐   C ☐

Suspected diagnosis:
Otitis Media with Effusion ☐   Normal tm ☐
                                   Abnormal tm ☐   Grade: ....

Sensorineural ☐   Confirmed ☐
                      Suspected ☐

Chronic Otitis Media ☐   Tubotympanic ☐
                             Attico-antral ☐

Management	
Visit	**Action**

Decision Indications for grommets	
Bilateral hearing loss of > 25db (or equivalent free field levels)	☐
Uncomplicated persisting > 3 months Supported by abnormal tympanogram	☐
Persisting significant Tympanic Membrane abnormality	☐
Otalgia	☐
Investigating Cochlea Function	☐
Recurrent Acute Otitis Media (> 6 months)	☐

Signature of Doctor: ....

Print name: ....

Page 6.

Figure 7.3 *(continued)*

m The Doncaster Royal
& Montagu Hospital

ADMISSION OF ENT PATIENTS

Unit Number...

Surname...

Forename(s)..

Date: .... Contact telephone number: ....

Consultant: ....

Date placed on waiting list: ....

Dates to avoid: ....

Intended Operation:

....

....

....

....

....

Clinical Priority:

Urgent	☐	
Soon	☐	
Routine	☐	
Dated:		

Operating Surgeon:

Cons	☐
S. Reg	☐
Reg	☐
Any	☐

Pre-clerking assessment:

Nurse led	☐
SHO	☐
To be done on admission	☐
Pre-admission completed	☐

Anaesthetic / Theatre highlights:

1. ....

2. ....

3. ....

4. ....

Instructions for Pre-op assessment

1. ....

2. ....

3. ....

4. ....

Admission instructions:

GA   DC   INP   LA   HYPNOVEL

Instructions on admission:

1. ....

2. ....

3. ....

4. ....

Consented: No / Yes

Information sheet given: No / Yes

Complications mentioned: No / Yes

Page 7.   Signature of Doctor: ....   Print name: ....

Figure 7.3 (*continued*)

Physical Examination

Weight: .... Kg

Pulse: .... / min   BP: .... / .... mm Hg

Heart Rhythm : Regular / Irregular   Heart Sounds: ....

Chest: Clear / Abnormal   Specify: ....

Cervical Spine or Dental Abnormalities   Yes / No

Specify: ....

Any other relevant factors: ....

E.N.T. Examination

Ears: (R)   (L)   Tuning Fork (512 Hz)

                                                (R)   (L)

                                                R

                                                W

Nose   Internal   External

                                Deviated ?

            PNS   Scars ?

Oropharynx   Larynx

Neck

Investigations	Performed			Abnormal	
	Yes	No		Yes	No
Full Blood Count	☐	☐		☐	☐
Urea / Electrolytes	☐	☐		☐	☐
Group and Save	☐	☐		☐	☐
Chest X-ray	☐	☐		☐	☐
Sinus X-ray	☐	☐		☐	☐
Electrocardiogram	☐	☐		☐	☐
Other:	☐	☐		☐	☐

CONSENT   Yes / No

Complications mentioned: ....

Signature: ....

Page 8.

Figure 7.3 (*continued*)

The Doncaster Royal
& Montagu Hospital

ENT ASSESSMENT

Unit Number..

Surname...

Forename(s)...

Date: ....   Day Case / In-patient   Planned / Emergency

Reason for admission: ....

....

....

Medical History

	Yes	No		Yes	No
Heart Disease / Angina	☐	☐	Hypertension	☐	☐
Bronchitis / Asthma	☐	☐	Diabetes Mellitus	☐	☐
Rheumatoid Arthritis	☐	☐	Epilepsy	☐	☐
Bleeding tendency	☐	☐	Possible Pregnancy	☐	☐
Other medical condition	☐	☐			

Give details: ....

....

....

Smoking: ....   Alcohol: ....

Medication: ....

Allergy: ....

Tympanogram required if the last test was > 4 weeks ago.

Date of last tympanogram: ....

Tympanogram required ?   Yes ☐   No ☐

Tympanogram carried out ? Yes ☐   No ☐

Anaesthetic History

	Yes	No	
Previous anaesthetic (If Yes, specify any problems)	☐	☐	
Family history of anaesthetic problems or reactions	☐	☐	
Cervical spine / jaw problems	☐	☐	
Teeth: Crowns / caps / loose teeth	☐	☐	
Sickle test required ?	☐	☐	
Intubation difficulties foreseen ?	☐	☐	

Page 9.

Figure 7.3 (*continued*)

The Doncaster Royal & Montagu Hospital

ADMISSION

Unit Number.................................... D.o.B. ....

Surname..

Forename(s)..

Date: ....

Details above checked and correct ? Yes / No

Name of Legal Guardian: ....

Address: ....

.... Telephone No.: ....

Child likes to be called: .... Age: .... Religion:....................

Consultant: .... G.P.: ....

Health Visitor / School Nurse / Social Worker: ....

Nursery / School: ....

Other Children: ....

Parent plans to be residential? Yes / No

Allergies?   No / Yes: State: ....

Current medication: ....

....

Handed to nurse Yes / No

Previous Medical / Surgical History: ....

....

Reason for admission: ....

Additional information: ....

....

....

....

Transport home discussed: ....

Is there anything special / specific we need to know to enable us to care for your child ?

Name of Admitting Nurse: ....

Signature: ....

Page 10.

Figure 7.3 (*continued*)

m The Doncaster Royal
& Montagu Hospital

ADL ASSESSMENT

Unit Number...

Surname...

Forename(s)...

I have no concerns over the following:

Nurses signature: ....   Parent signature: ....

Usual Pattern (Self / Family Care)	Alterations caused by illness / admission and presentation
Breathing and circulation	
Red Book	
Safety	
Food and drink	
Cultural and religious observations	
Play and activity	
Communication	
Comfort, rest and sleep	
Hygiene	
Elimination	
Mobility	
Maintain body temperature	
Expressing sexuality	

Comments:

Page 11.

Figure 7.3 (*continued*)

The Doncaster Royal
& Montagu Hospital

ADMISSION DAY

Unit Number...

Surname...

Forename(s)..

Date: .... Time of admission: .... Planned theatre time: ....

Nursing:

		Yes	N/A	
1.	Welcome to ward	☐	☐	....
2.	Introduction to Named Nurse:	☐	☐	....
3.	Commence patient assessment (within 12 hours of admission)	☐	☐	....
4.	Record temperature, pulse, respirations, blood pressure and pain score	☐	☐	....
5.	Record weight: .... kg	☐	☐	....
6.	Explain pre- and post-operative procedures	☐	☐	....
7.	Has anything changed since the child was pre-clerked ? (state below)	☐	☐	....
8.	Discuss questions	☐	☐	....
	a. Last hearing test: .... / .... /	☐	☐	....
	b. Last tympanogram: .... / .... /	☐	☐	....
9.	Give reassurance regarding anxieties	☐	☐	....
10.	Assess and record Dependence Score on computer	☐	☐	....
11.	Assess moving and handling risk	☐	☐	....
12.	Assess and record Waterlow Score:	☐	☐	....
13.	Orientate child and family to ward and team	☐	☐	....
14.	Commence discharge planning	☐	☐	....

Pre-Op Care:

		Yes	N/A	
15.	Complete Ward Check-list (on back of consent)	☐	☐	....
16.	Choice of gown	☐	☐	....
17.	Choice of transport	☐	☐	....
18.	Escort to anaesthetic room	☐	☐	....
19.	Stay with child until anaesthetised	☐	☐	....
20.	Escort parent(s) back to ward and give reassurance	☐	☐	....
	Note any variables	☐	☐	

Print Name: .... Signed (Early Shift): ....

Print Name: .... Signed (Late Shift): ....

Multidisciplinary Continuation Sheet		
Time	Variables / Continuation of Notes	Signature/Profession

Page 12.

Figure 7.3 (*continued*)

m The Doncaster Royal & Montagu Hospital		*AFFIX LABEL HERE IF AVAILABLE*	
		Unit Number...	
		Surname...	
THEATRE		Forename(s)...	

Date: ....

		Yes	No	
1.	Check identity verbally with patient / relative / escort	☐	☐	....
2.	Check notes and consent completed	☐	☐	....
3.	Position on operating table / trolley:	☐	☐	....
4.	Pressure relieving device used	☐	☐	....
5.	Swab count correct	☐	☐	....
6.	Instrument count correct	☐	☐	....
Note any variables		☐	☐	....

Print Name: .... Signed: ....

	Multidisciplinary Continuation Sheet	
Time	Variables	Signature/Profession
	Continuation of Notes	
Time		Signature/Profession

Page 13.

Figure 7.3 (*continued*)

Theatre Use Only
Insert Theatre Check-list here

Figure 7.3 (*continued*)

	AFFIX LABEL HERE IF AVAILABLE
m The Doncaster Royal & Montagu Hospital	Unit Number..
	Surname..
RETURN TO WARD	Forename(s)...

Date: ....

Nursing: **Yes   N/A**

1. Receive hand-over from recovery staff on ward ☐ ☐ ....
2. Ensure safe transfer to bed ☐ ☐ ....
3. Position in bed correctly, cot sides as appropriate ☐ ☐ ....
4. Record post-op observations as per protocol ☐ ☐ ....
5. Observe cannula site for pain, redness, leakage or swelling ☐ ☐ ....
6. Assess pain using chart ☐ ☐ ....
7. Give analgesia as required ☐ ☐ ....
8. Observe for aural loss ☐ ☐ ....
9. Maintain dressing ☐ ☐ ....
10. Administer ear-drops as prescribed ☐ ☐ ....
11. Maintain IVI in situ ☐ ☐ ....
12. Offer fluids and diet as tolerated ☐ ☐ ....
13. Passed urine ☐ ☐ ....

Specific additional care:

1. Observe for excessive swallowing ☐ ☐ ....
2. Observe for oral loss ☐ ☐ ....
3. Observe for nasal loss ☐ ☐ ....
4. Observe facial nerve ☐ ☐ ....
5. Maintain pressure bandage ☐ ☐ ....
Note any variables ☐

Print Name: .... Signed (Early Shift): ....

Print Name: .... Signed (Late Shift): ....

Print Name: .... Signed (Night Shift): ....

POST-OPERATIVE DAY 1

Date: ....

Nursing: **Yes   N/A**

1. Assist with hygiene by: .... ☐ ☐ ....
2. Remove IVI if in situ ☐ ☐ ....
3. Assess pain; give analgesia as required ☐ ☐ ....
4. Record observations as per protocol ☐ ☐ ....
5. Remove dressing(s) if in situ ☐ ☐ ....
6. Ensure diet and fluids are tolerated ☐ ☐ ....
   Note any variables

Print Name: .... Signed (Early Shift): ....

Print Name: .... Signed (Late Shift): ....

Page 14.

Figure 7.3 (*continued*)

	The Doncaster Royal & Montagu Hospital	*AFFIX LABEL HERE IF AVAILABLE*	
		Unit Number...	
		Surname..	
	CONTINUATION NOTES	Forename(s)...	

	Multidisciplinary Continuation Sheet		
Time	Variables	Signature/Profession	
Time	Continuation of Notes	Signature/Profession	

Page 15.

Figure 7.3 (*continued*)

m The Doncaster Royal
& Montagu Hospital

DISCHARGE

AFFIX LABEL HERE IF AVAILABLE

Unit Number...

Surname...

Forename(s)..

Date: .... Time of discharge for patient / family: ....

Nursing:

		Yes	N/A
1.	Discharge according to plan	☐	☐
2.	Remove IV cannula / sub-cut cannula	☐	☐
3.	Ensure legal guardians have advice leaflets	☐	☐
4.	Ensure TTO's prescribed and given	☐	☐
5.	Give parent out-patient appointment	☐	☐ To be sent ☐
6.	Give parent hearing test appointment	☐	☐
7.	Ensure discharge letter is complete	☐	☐
	Copy to GP	☐	☐
	Copy to Health Visitor Liaison	☐	☐

Note any variables ☐

Print Name: .... Signed: ....

Multidisciplinary Continuation Sheet

Time	Variables	Signature/Profession

Time	Continuation of Notes	Signature/Profession

Page 16.

Figure 7.3 (*continued*)

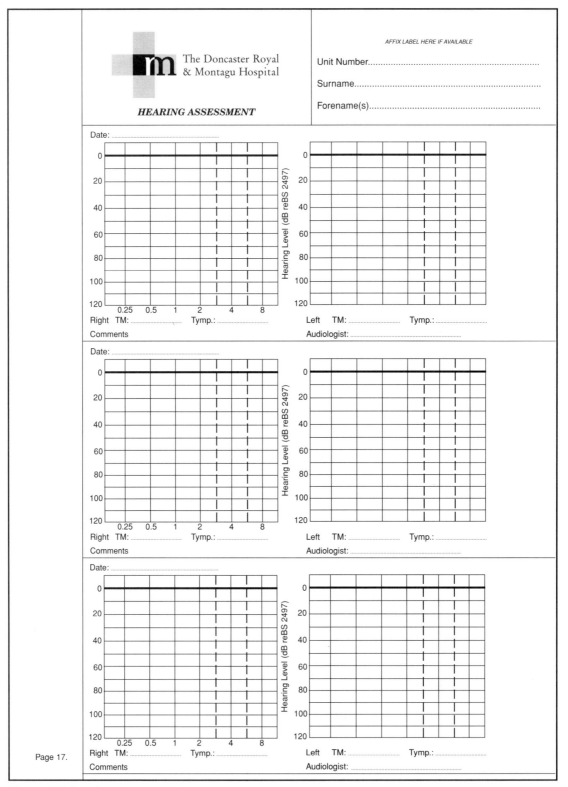

Figure 7.3 (*continued*)

m The Doncaster Royal & Montagu Hospital	*AFFIX LABEL HERE IF AVAILABLE* Unit Number.. Surname.. Forename(s)...
HEARING ASSESSMENT	

Date: ....

Warble 0.5KHz	Warble 0.5KHz
Warble 2KHz	Warble 2KHz
Warble 4KHz	Warble 4KHz
High freq. rattle	High freq. rattle
Location	Location
Other	Other

Right   TM .... Tymp: ....   Left   TM .... Tymp: ....

Comments: Audiologist: ....

Date: ....

Warble 0.5KHz	Warble 0.5KHz
Warble 2KHz	Warble 2KHz
Warble 4KHz	Warble 4KHz
High freq. rattle	High freq. rattle
Location	Location
Other	Other

Right   TM .... Tymp: ....   Left   TM .... Tymp: ....

Comments: Audiologist: ....

Date: ....

Warble 0.5KHz	Warble 0.5KHz
Warble 2KHz	Warble 2KHz
Warble 4KHz	Warble 4KHz
High freq. rattle	High freq. rattle
Location	Location
Other	Other

Right   TM .... Tymp: ....   Left   TM .... Tymp: ....

Comments: Audiologist: ....

Additional Comments:

Figure 7.3 (*continued*)

AUDIT TRAIL	AFFIX LABEL HERE IF AVAILABLE Unit Number.. Surname... Forename(s)...

To be completed on Discharge or move to Major Ear Surgery

Date of completion: .... / .... / ....   Discharge ☐   Major Ear Surgery ☐

	Yes	No	
Tympanic membrane damage	☐	☐	....
Atelectasis	☐	☐	....
Tympanosclerosis	☐	☐	....
Perforation	☐	☐	....
SN Loss	☐	☐	....
Number of grommet insertions	☐	☐	....
Aenoidectomy	☐	☐	....
Complications during treatment	☐	☐	....
Otitis Media	☐	☐	....
Other	☐	☐	....
Ototoxic ear drops used	☐	☐	....
Major ear surgery needed	☐	☐	....
Mastoidectomy	☐	☐	....
Myringoplasty	☐	☐	....
Tympanoplasty	☐	☐	....
Ossiculoplasty	☐	☐	....
CAT	☐	☐	....

Other relevant comments:

Signature: ....   Print Name: ....

Return this sheet to:

Tracy P. Evans, IPOC Co-ordinator,
Department of Clinical Audit, Research & Effectiveness

Page 19.

Figure 7.3 (*continued*)

8

Maintaining momentum

Rhona Hotchkiss

Introduction

In keeping with other change management initiatives, the successful development and implementation of ICPs requires careful planning and effective project management. Realistically, it is important to be aware that some ICPs fail and success is not always guaranteed. Steps can be taken, however, to greatly increase the chances of success. Time and effort must be spent in preparing the ground for change, in managing the expectations of staff in terms of timescale and potential benefits and in developing strategies to maintain momentum once the change process has begun.

This chapter explores these themes in more detail with a particular emphasis on establishing and 'maintaining momentum'.

Preparing the main players

The facilitator

Usually, although not always or necessarily from a clinical background, the facilitator must be prepared to, and be capable of, operating on several different levels simultaneously. They will need the ability to work with:

- qualified and unqualified nursing staff
- clerical and ancillary staff
- peers from a range of clinical disciplines and professions
- senior/consultant level medical staff, and
- senior managers.

In addition, if ICPs are being developed in or in conjunction with community-based services, the facilitator will also work closely with a diverse range of professionals and staff from other agencies, e.g. social services.

In terms of accountability, facilitators may be answerable to and should be supervised and supported by the director of medicine or nursing, the chief executive or the local health care co-operative (LHCC)/primary care group (PCG)/local health group (LHG) leader.

It is also important that facilitators, particularly those developing ICPs for the first time, are aware that:

- Pathways are rarely an unqualified success at the first 'draft' stage.
- Their development can be protracted, stormy and tortuous and can involve a pattern of 'two steps forward, one step back'.
- The potential exists for pathways to 'fail' for a variety of reasons.

Why ICPs fail

Facilitators should be aware of the reasons why ICPs are not always a success and also understand that many of these reasons are no reflection on their own skills. In 'lone' posts, such as that of ICP facilitator, there is a temptation for the post-holder to view success and failure as an expression of their own competence; experience suggests that this is not the case. However, ICPs do fail for *avoidable* reasons and the facilitator should consider the following factors prior to commencing a pathway development project:

- ICPs are not a universal panacea and may not be the correct approach for the chosen condition, that clinical and managerial team or that clinical area; at present there are few pointers to help staff decide if their clinical area or any particular condition are amenable to the use of an ICP, but generally speaking surgical conditions seem more straightforward than do medical, hospital care more amenable than community-based situations and single pathology less complex than multi-pathology.

- There has to be a consensus amongst staff that this is how they wish to proceed, or at the very least that they are willing to try the pathways approach. The enthusiasm of one or two staff members will not be enough to carry the pathway through the months of development which lie ahead. As a general rule, more than half of the staff, including all of the senior staff, must be in favour or at least not actively opposed; more than a few dissenters will make change difficult to introduce or sustain.
- It is not uncommon for the impetus to develop ICPs to come largely from one professional group, with staff from that group remaining disproportionately involved and supportive. Whilst pathways can bring benefits to any one discipline through, for example, reduced and streamlined documentation or more accessible audit data, the potential for benefit is maximized when the entire clinical team is involved in both the introduction and ongoing development of pathways.

Why ICPs succeed

ICPs do, of course, succeed and facilitators can make their own task much easier by ensuring that those factors which can combine to make ICPs a success are incorporated into the project design from its beginning.

The day-to-day success of ICPs, particularly in a hospital ward setting, will depend to a very large extent on the ward manager. If the impetus to develop ICPs has not actually come from the ward manager, they must at the very least be fully committed to the project and prepared to play an active part in its introduction and development. They should accept responsibility for:

- using the pathway themselves;
- ensuring that other nursing staff use it;
- encouraging junior medical staff to use it.

The ultimate success or failure of ICPs is arguably dependent on the involvement and support of consultant medical staff. If they help develop the documentation, refer to or record in it daily, offer feedback on its use and contribute to its refinement, junior medical staff are likely to follow suit. If the consultant

does not become involved in this way, it will almost certainly fail as a multidisciplinary project.

The facilitator's most crucial task in the initial pre-development stage of introducing ICPs arguably lies in persuading senior medical staff to give ICPs a chance. It is difficult to introduce ICPs to an area on a partial basis, that is for the patients of one consultant but not another – the situation simply becomes too confusing for staff and for patients.

Clinical staff

Facilitators have to be able to deal with and counter difficulties staff have with the concept of ICPs as they arise. Most of the queries and objections are common ones and have been dealt with in other articles (Hotchkiss, 1997). In particular though, medical staff can have difficulty with the concept of pre-printed documentation. Medical staff are in the main, accustomed to approaching patients to take a history, make an operation note or contribute to progress notes armed only with a blank sheet of paper. The very laudable argument goes that every patient is an individual and things are not done in medicine to a recipe. Facilitators would do well to arm themselves with data from audits of existing case notes, which time and again demonstrate that this is not the case and which will invariably underline the highly stylized and repetitive nature of medical documentation.

The facilitator might also suggest to consultant medical staff that ICPs are not 'for' them, given that they do very little of the routine documentation on most patients. They are, however, 'for' them in that they are one way of ensuring that junior medical staff both provide and document care in the manner that consultants wish and furthermore are a way of ensuring that particular and even 'routine' tasks, tests and investigations are not missed.

The most important point to stress to senior medical staff is that ICPs are not intended and should not be designed either in format or content to limit individual clinical judgement. Where clinical judgement equates to the ability to do what is appropriate for an individual in any situation, ICPs are and should be no barrier. If consultants are fully involved in the design and implementation, the content will in any case, be to their specification and alterations made at their direction.

The popular maxim, 'if it ain't broke, don't fix it' is applied in health care as much as anywhere else in life and to documentation as much as to any other task or procedure. The facilitator will have to demonstrate that:

- it is broke;
- it has the potential to break;
- it ain't broke, but we could make it work better.

Any one of the above approaches might be employed and they are not listed in any particular order of frequency. A quick glance through the Health Commissioner's reports for any one year will demonstrate how, on numerous occasions, health professionals thought their documentation adequate, when clearly it was not. A further useful exercise might be to measure documentation *in its completed form* against the relevant King's Fund standards on documentation. Alternatively, a useful if somewhat pedantic way of demonstrating how the situation could be improved is simply to count the number of times that the same information, for example demographic information on admission, is recorded for one patient. This is at best a situation which means information being laboriously hand copied from one part of the record to the other, and, at worst, sees the patient being asked the same questions time and time again.

In order for staff, especially senior staff, to embrace change, there will have to be some appreciable benefit to themselves or to their patients. Potential and actual benefits from the introduction of pathways are increasingly being documented and facilitators should be aware of these. However, it is enormously important to stress to staff at this stage, that many of the expected benefits are of a potential nature only, and until the document is refined enough to be used without ongoing major changes in its structure or content, they will not be realized in full. At this stage, it may also be appropriate to highlight the immediate benefits which can be realized prior to implementation of ICPs, namely that:

- current practice is reviewed;
- the individual roles of each member of the clinical team are clearly defined;

- collaboration and communication between members of the clinical team can be improved;
- the aims and objectives of providing care to the chosen client group are reinforced.

Clinical audit/clinical effectiveness
The potential for ICP documentation to capture data for audit in a form which is easily retrieved and understood makes their use an attractive proposition. In many organizations, they have been introduced at the instigation or under the auspices of the clinical audit department. Health service staff face a baffling array of new information about clinically effective care on an ongoing basis. As a result, one of the most difficult tasks facing audit/effectiveness staff is in discovering ways to get information to frontline health care professionals, and to find ways to encourage its incorporation into everyday practice. A new clinical guideline, no matter how demonstrably evidence based, may never make the successful transition from publication to practice. Documentation which reminds staff of the requirements of a new guideline, e.g. assessing patient need for deep venous thrombosis prophylaxis, in a form which requires them to carry out a specified task or to document the reasons why they have not done so, may ease that necessary transition.

Before the ICP is used in practice, the facilitator should encourage staff to identify priorities for audit. The amount of information produced from the use of ICP documentation is potentially overwhelming, and any attempt to utilize all of it will leave people overwhelmed and frustrated!

In terms of managing expectations, it is important that the length of time and effort required to get the pathway to a 'usable' and relatively 'stable' state is not underestimated. This is the most vital step the facilitator can take in preventing de-motivation of participating staff. There is also a strong temptation for ICP facilitators, convinced of the worth and potential of pathways, to overstate their case and even to make unrealistic claims about the capacity of ICPs to deliver change and improvement. It is better in motivational terms to understate potential and see expectations realized and then exceeded, than to have staff frustrated and disappointed when their efforts do not realize the anticipated rewards.

ICPs are not a quick fix. Project timetables covering a few weeks are entirely unrealistic and if staff appreciate from the beginning that the refining process may occur over a number of months, they may not so readily abandon the project if it does not deliver immediate rewards.

Managerial staff

A critical success factor for the introduction of ICPs is the 'top-down' support of senior management. There needs to be a tangible commitment of resources to support the initiative, which will require time for all its benefits to be realized, e.g. establishing 'absolute' value for money. The resources required to get an ICP project underway are not inconsiderable. At the very least it will involve:

- a full-time or designated facilitator;
- office space;
- IT and reproduction facilities;
- time for clinical staff to participate in designing and reviewing the pathway.

Introducing, producing and supporting pathways is essentially a full-time job. It is not a task that can be easily added to the existing responsibilities of an existing member of staff, particularly if the main responsibilities of the post include:

- base-line audits of documentation and practice;
- discussions with all key staff;
- education sessions with all clinical staff (including night staff);
- production and continuing refinement of the documentation.

The facilitator will have to be sufficiently experienced and confident enough to work with the various participants and should be remunerated at a level which suggests that the organization places some value on ICP development.

In addition to having a base from which to work, the facilitator will require or should have access to skills and facilities that will allow them to produce a standard of documentation that staff will want to use. ICP layout and content can change very frequently, particularly in the initial stages, even if only in minor detail. Having ICPs printed in large numbers when they have passed the initial

development stages is inadvisable. Pathway documentation is intended to be dynamic – it should change from time to time as new guidelines and updated practices are taken on board. One of the selling points for the introduction of an ICP documentation system is the move away from the practice of using the same documentation without regard to changes in care or treatment for long periods of time, or generic documentation for all admissions to hospital or other care settings. If pathway documentation becomes as stagnant and non-dynamic as the system it replaces, it loses one of its main attractions.

Facilitators must have the ability, the capacity and the resources to make changes to documentation as and when clinical staff identify a deficit. A speedy response should minimize the opportunity for staff to develop a negative attitude to the documentation, or indeed for any untoward incident to occur in terms of the delivery or documentation of patient care. The production and reproduction of documentation can be extremely time consuming. The more inclusive and therefore inherently complex the pathway is, the more it is likely to require adjustments on an ongoing basis. A minor point, but one of some importance in the production/reproduction scenario, is the use of pathways that incorporate different coloured sections for different stages of care. This can be very helpful in terms of helping people locate and retrieve particular pieces of data, but a further complicating factor for the in-house production of documentation.

Keeping up the momentum

Having taken the ICP to implementation stage, the facilitator and the clinical team now face a further set of potential hurdles and difficulties. Included within this are:

- insufficient time away from direct patient care for staff to familiarize themselves with and ask questions about new documentation;
- a perception that ICP documentation takes longer to complete and requires more writing;
- the inevitability that inadequacies in new documentation will only become clear with use.

Insufficient time

Staff in clinical areas rarely have 'protected' time to spend away from their normal day-to-day duties poring over new documentation and becoming familiar with it. For this reason, the most determined facilitator in operation will probably not be able to explain the ICP to all staff on a 'one-to-one' basis. Verbal advice and information should therefore be supported by written information provided for all staff, perhaps in the form of a laminated pocket-sized 'how to use ICPs' guide, complete with contact numbers and names of staff who can offer advice and assistance when difficulties arise.

Perceptions about documentation

Staff may suggest that the ICP documentation takes longer to complete than did the existing system of documentation and this may well be accurate. However, the documentation is likely to take more time to complete for one of two reasons, neither of which is likely to continue in the long term:

1 Any new system requires familiarization time. The act of having to turn pages over to find where to document a particular piece of information rather than simply writing it down on the next piece of blank paper will be more time consuming until staff are able to turn to the required place automatically.
2 ICPs may actually require some staff to write more than they did before, particularly in situations where previous documentation was not well completed and where 'routine' notes about patients' progress were not kept to an adequate standard. Properly designed pathway documentation *can not* require staff to write more, if they were already documenting at a satisfactorily safe level. ICP documentation is concerned with anticipating the 'routine' of clinical record keeping and pre-printing it, thus allowing the clinician to follow or not follow what was anticipated. However, practical experience has shown, that staff – especially those who may have been at best ambivalent about the introduction of ICPs – sometimes perceive them to be an added administrative burden. It may take a word count by the facilitator, of records, pre and post ICPs, to demonstrate that this is not the case and that in most instances, lack of familiarity with the documentation promotes these negative perceptions.

Inadequacies in the new documentation

Even with the best efforts of enthusiastic staff from all disciplines involved, ICPs will always require changes to be made following implementation. The need for changes due to the emergence of new guidelines or changes in practice has been highlighted earlier in this chapter. In addition, the pilot phase of implementation will reveal inadequacies in the new documentation that will also require change. The facilitator must prepare staff for this actuality to avoid their becoming de-motivated. However, it is advisable to leave these changes until the pilot phase is completed unless a dangerous or obvious omission is recognized. Too many changes during an ongoing pilot provides the potential to confuse or frustrate the staff involved.

Communicating success

In terms of maintaining momentum, the most successful motivating factor for the facilitator and for staff, is the ability to demonstrate success. Once the ICP is in use, routine monitoring may highlight an improvement in patient outcomes or reductions in length of stay and it is important that the benefits achieved through pathway use are shared with the staff involved and to staff in other clinical areas. Sharing success in this manner reinforces the use of ICPs within the organization and may also help to encourage more reluctant peers to become involved in the next phase of ICP development. A key factor in this process is analysis of variations from the expected and its role in reflective practice. In particular, the staff involved in using the pathway may have identified priorities for audit made possible by the ICP. In these cases, the facilitator must take responsibility for compiling the information and seeing the process through to a stage where staff are either re-assured about their practice or necessary changes are agreed and incorporated into the pathway.

The longer term

The longer an ICP is in place, the greater chance it has of becoming established and accepted practice. New staff join the team, unaware that any other way of working existed previously; newly qualified staff from all disciplines – often more open to new ways of working – join the team or pass through the area and begin to spread the word about the usefulness of ICPs. However, even pathways that have been in place for in advance of a year can be discontinued, for any of the reasons already stated. The facilitator and the clinicians involved will have to examine their own practice and their part, if any, in the failure of the ICP. What facilitators must never do, is blame themselves completely, or become so discouraged they never again get involved in the introduction of ICPs.

Working in this project management-type role is potentially a very isolating experience; facilitators should make every effort to share responsibility, concerns and success with the local clinical teams and should also look outwards to supportive networks which might exist.

Conclusion

Maintaining momentum with ICPs can be seen as the balance of four factors, namely:

- Preparing the ground – identifying an appropriate topic and clinic area, establishing support from senior clinical staff.
- Good project management – including realistic expectations in terms of timescale(s) and the potential benefits for both staff and patients.
- Determination – on behalf of the project facilitator and other key players to see the project through to completion.
- Learning from failure and communicating success throughout the organization.

The facilitator also has a responsibility for devolving their expertise to others working with them which will help to ensure momentum is maintained if they move or find that the nature of the role precludes them from participating in every ICP project.

Reference

Hotchkiss, R. (1997) Managing care: integrated care pathways. *Research*, 2(1), 30–36.

9

Evaluating care pathways

Kathryn de Luc

Introduction

In this era of evidence-based practice in health care, it is right for organizations to question the effectiveness of ICPs before they commit their own resources for their long-term development and use. Whilst, as yet, no comprehensive clinical and/or cost effectiveness analyses of pathways has been published in the UK, the fact that they take time and resources to develop is already well recognized (Del Togno-Armanasco et al., 1993 p.137; Greengold and Weingarten, 1996; Holtzman et al., 1998; Tonges and Brett, 1995 p.177).

This chapter provides practical advice as to how you might evaluate the ICPs introduced in your own organization.

What do we mean by evaluation?

It is important to define what is meant by evaluation. Hale (1997 p.288) has highlighted both ends of the spectrum when interpreting the term. The first concerns the 'common sense' usage involving a personal judgement/assessment as to the worth of a particular intervention. In contrast, a second interpretation is used in the research literature and this refers to a particular research approach used to assess the effects of something, often an intervention or innovation. It does not require a particular research strategy, but can use the traditional experimental, survey or case study approaches (Robson, 1993 p.170) or some combination of them. When embarking on an evaluation, you will need to be clear about which kind of evaluation you want to carry out, and this in turn depends on its ultimate use. 'Fit for purpose' is the key

phrasing which needs to be borne in mind. Both types of evaluation are equally valid for a particular purpose, and in order to decide which approach to take you need to identify for what purpose the evaluation is going to be used.

The next section of this chapter looks at some of the issues you are likely to face if you intend to undertake an evaluation study. Some of these issues will be applicable irrespective of whichever type of evaluation is planned, whereas others will be more relevant to a principally research-based evaluation study.

Local flexibility in the design of care pathways

One of the problems that has been identified in the literature surrounding pathways is the lack of a precise definition as to what a pathway is, and what it contains (de Luc and Currie, 1999; Hale, 1997 p.284; Shreifer, 1994). This means that there is no standardization of the tool: many studies are using slightly different definitions and interpretations. There is some tentative evidence that different ICP models are operating within the UK (de Luc and Currie, 1999), which in turn represent different primary functions. For example some pathways are aimed at achieving a more patient-focused service, whilst others place greater emphasis on clinical effectiveness. It seems likely that differences in primary functions will result in different designs of pathways and therefore different outcomes. It is essential therefore when evaluating the effectiveness of the introduction of ICPs to clarify and document both the objectives for the pathway under evaluation and the elements included within the pathway.

Deciding what to measure – the focus of your evaluation

Two key questions you may want to ask are 'how do we know if the ICP has made a difference?' and if so, 'precisely what difference has it made?' These questions can involve the measurement of outcomes at the patient, individual clinical staff, clinical team and at the organizational level (e.g. trust, PCG). Examples of outcomes that can be measured include:

- patients including clinical outcomes, satisfaction levels and patient education/ knowledge about the condition and self-management, etc.;
- individual clinical staff delivering the care, e.g. job satisfaction, staff turnover, morale and stress levels;
- the clinical team developing and designing the pathway, e.g. increased multidisciplinary working, system changes in the way care is delivered, use of the pathway documentation, development of local protocols/guidelines, communication improvements, risk management, etc.;
- organizational outcomes, e.g. promotion of continuous quality improvement ethos, implementation of evidence-based practice, efficiency improvements, increased provision of integrated care, an improved model with which to cost care, etc.

The key is to decide the focus of your evaluation and the features you therefore wish to measure. For example, do you want to measure the effect of one particular pathway on the care delivered? If so, you probably will want to concentrate at the patient, individual clinician and at the clinical team levels of outcome monitoring. On the other hand, if you are reviewing the effect of pathways per se on an organization you might think about looking at more than one pathway and its effect. In this instance, the outcome evaluation will be at the organizational as well as at the individual level. To date, few, if any, evaluations in the UK have been done at this organizational level, because few organizations have sufficient pathways in operation to effect organization wide change.

You need to decide at the outset the focus of your evaluation and what kind of outcomes you are going to measure.

Evaluation of a single pathway

If you undertake an evaluation of a single pathway, then you need to decide which aspect(s) of the pathway you wish to measure. ICPs are multi-faceted tools: they comprise a number of different elements and have the primary purpose of supporting clinical processes. One way of distinguishing these different elements is to differentiate between the development and the operation of the ICP.

During the development of ICPs, pathways act as an agent for change. This (first) aspect concentrates on issues of cultural change, which surround the development of multidisciplinary working, streamlining the process of care, agreeing standards of clinical communication and putting evidence and guidelines into practice. The second aspect is how ICPs operate to deliver patient care. This involves using the pathway as a mechanism for the clinical management of individual patients, which, in turn, allows the aggregation of results for auditing and monitoring purposes.

Table 9.1 Possible areas to examine

- Changes in clinical documentation resulting from introduction of pathway template.
- Accuracy/completeness and/or amount of time to complete.
- Changes in clinical care, e.g. introduction of guidelines, increased consistency in care, changes in process of care delivery, e.g. length of stay, shortening time delays in the process, reducing number of visits, changes in who does what.
- Changes in patient satisfaction.
- Effect of patient education/information on the knowledge the patient has.
- Changes in clinical outcomes.
- Views of staff on introduction of pathways.
- Quality of life changes for the patient.
- Effect on clinical team providing the care, e.g. team building, multidisciplinary working, job satisfaction.
- Effect of variance reporting.
- Cost analysis or cost benefit analysis.
- Effect of computerization of pathways.

Evaluation of multiple pathways

If you are evaluating multiple pathways then the potential to compare the effects of different pathways exists. If different elements or design features exist across a range of pathways, then these can be compared, as can the development process used to develop the pathways if different processes were employed. This type of comparison would provide some evidence as to which features work best in an ICP and why.

Designing the evaluation

There are many different types of evaluation. The choice of which design should be determined by the aspect of ICPs you wish to examine. The three most common strategies are:

- experiment
- survey
- case study.

Another strategy commonly considered when evaluating ICPs is:

- participatory action research.

These approaches are briefly outlined here in the context of evaluating ICPs. Each design has its strengths and weaknesses that, together with full descriptions of the approaches, can be found in the research literature.

Experimental and quasi-experimental designs

The number of experimental or quasi-experimental published studies of ICPs is limited. In the randomized control trial (RCT), participants are allocated at random to receive two or more forms of care. In the context of pathways this may be two or more groups of patients receiving care for a particular condition, one group on the pathway and the other not. The point is that the patients who are measured are assigned to one or the other of the groups at random. In the literature on ICPs there are a few studies reported which state they have used an RCT methodology (Dowsey et al., 1999; Falconer et al., 1993).

The non-RCT experiment and quasi-experimental approach has many variations, but essentially involves some form of experimental or study group being compared to some form of control group. The participants of both groups are not randomly assigned, and the collection of the data takes place usually simultaneously in both groups. The difficulty with these approaches and similarly with RCTs is that they are complicated to set up in the context of a busy hospital/GP surgery. For

example, to get the same staff to use two different clinical documentation systems (the pathway and original documentation) is not easy. Likewise, using two different locations is equally difficult to control, with the added complication of ensuring that there are no other differences between the locations, which may affect the results. Because of these difficulties, the before-and-after-study design, where the collection of data is made sequentially from the two groups being compared, is the most frequently used to study ICPs (Bailey et al., 1998; Cannon et al., 1999; Hofmann, 1993; Holtzman et al., 1998; Huber et al., 1998; Kwan-Gett et al., 1997; Riley, 1999; Wright et al., 1997).

Surveys

Surveys are used to make inferences about a large group of people from data drawn from a relatively small number of individuals within that group. This method has been usefully employed when data needs to be collected in a relatively small and specific area that can be pre-determined with the use of specific questions. The results can be generalized to a larger population and, with the application of statistical methods, can identify the limits of error. To date survey approaches have been used to examine a number of aspects of ICPs and these include patient clinical outcomes, e.g. quality of life measurements, patient satisfaction, patient education, and staff and patient views on the use of pathways.

Some studies have already been completed involving semi-structured interviews of staff from a number of organizations to obtain their views on the development of ICPs (Parsley, 1998; Riley, 1999; Taylor, 1997). In addition, surveys have been completed to determine the extent of ICP usage (Riley, 1998; Currie, 1999).

Surveys can be a very useful tool in the evaluation of ICPs because they can be used to collect a wide range of different types of information. They tend to produce information that is less detailed than case studies or action research approaches but they can be applied over a broad area.

Case studies

Case studies are often employed when studying a complex intervention in a real life context, where the factors under examination cannot be fully pre-determined and where there is no clear set of outcomes. This approach is often used in a more exploratory study where an in-depth approach is needed. In the context of ICPs, the focus of the study can be on a particular organization, a particular clinical team, or on a particular group of patients. This approach has also been used to focus on the process of change as the pathway is developed and implemented (Brown and Simpson, 1994; Council of International Hospitals, 1993a, 1993b; Gibb and Banfield, 1996; Gibb et al., 1995; Riley, 1999).

Case studies enable an in-depth and flexible analysis within natural surroundings and which are not artificially drawn up. They provide a real world setting that can make it easier for the audience of the evaluation to relate to and identify with.

Participatory action research

This is a term coined by Lewin (1946) and is similar to the case study approach. However, it accepts as valid and reliable the involvement of the person doing the research in the intervention being evaluated and usually does not involve an 'outside' researcher coming into the organization specifically to carry out the evaluation. It consists of planning the intervention, the implementation of the intervention, observing what happens, and ultimately in the context of pathways, adapting the pathway based on the observations and reflections made during the process. Participatory action research has received criticism from those who favour a more scientific approach, but it has been very useful in discovering and reflecting on interventions that have concentrated on the process of change within organizations. Robson (1993 p.442) provides a concise review of the criticisms and advantages of the action research approach. It is an approach that has been applied to ICPs, particularly in descriptive studies where the same person appears to have acted as the pathway facilitator as well as reporting the effects of using the pathway (Gibb and Banfield, 1996). In particular the approach has been used most effectively in providing valuable insights into the complex issues surrounding the development and implementation of ICPs.

Basis for comparison

One of the issues that has limited the number of evaluations undertaken to date is the necessity to collect some baseline or control information. The old adage that you don't know how far you have moved unless you know where you started applies here. It is as relevant to a study which examines the clinical care provided as it is to a study which involves an examination of the variations reported from the use of the pathway. The same can be said of examining the effect on patient satisfaction, the development of multidisciplinary teams and new documentation. Unfortunately, there is no shortcut if you want to evaluate the changes or outcomes achieved by the use of an ICP.

The problem is not so much that the information is not there, but rather one of time and resources to collect or extract the baseline or control information. Depending on what type of information you are collecting, that information may be sitting in medical records, it may be on a computer system or, if it is opinion-based, it may require some form of survey or interview process to collect it. It is important to be realistic about what can be collected for a baseline review within the resources available. The tendency is to over-estimate the amount of information you will need for this purpose. It is also vital not to over-estimate the information that is available.

Assessment of any changes that may have occurred

In order to make an assessment of any changes that may have occurred, the following issues need to be borne in mind.

1. Sample size

Dependent on the type of evaluation you wish to undertake, consideration needs to be given to the sample size required. This becomes particularly important if you are trying to measure changes that have occurred in (say) patient care or patient satisfaction as a result of using the pathway and if you intend to undertake some statistical analysis to measure such changes. Many of the evaluation studies completed to date suffer from the problem of small sample sizes (usually between 50 to 100). Kwan-Gett et al.'s (1997) study of an in-patient asthma pathway is rare in that it had a sample size of almost 600 patients. The problem with a small sample size is that you cannot be statistically confident that any changes which have occurred have happened due to the introduction of the ICP and not simply by chance. On the other hand, to get a large sample takes time. You need either to choose a pathway that has a considerable throughput of patients in a relatively short space of time or to consider using more than one site (be it hospital, GP practice, etc.) to increase the throughput of patients that can be measured.

In deciding the sample size you want to use, you need to think back to the purpose of your evaluation. Is this evaluation to make a personal judgement/assessment about the value of ICPs, or does it form part of a formal research proposal where it is planned to test for statistical significance any changes that may have occurred as a result of using the ICP? In the former scenario a relatively small sample size may suffice (20–30 cases); in the latter a much larger sample will be needed.

2. Validity

Internal validity is concerned with whether the changes measured are caused by the factor you are trying to measure (in this case the pathway) and not something else (usually called a 'confounder').

Some of the main issues affecting validity which need to be considered include:

• Initial differences in patient characteristics between the groups being compared (e.g. age, gender, severity of illness). This type of confounder is commonly dealt with in clinical studies with large sample sizes by using the matched pairs design. This involves identifying the variable that may be affecting the result and then identifying matched pairs of subjects who are then randomly assigned to the study group and control or baseline group (Robson, 1993 p.93).
• Initial differences in staff characteristics between the groups being compared. For example, whether there has been previous use of pathways and/or multidisciplinary documentation. If one's study involves

some collection of views and attitudes of staff to the introduction of a pathway, previous knowledge and experience of using these or other similar tools (whether positive or negative) will inevitably affect the responses. It is worth collecting this type of information so that you know your starting point.

• Local differences, e.g. different wards, variations in practices by individual doctors, nurses, etc. The use of standardized guidelines and protocols for the different locations or individual staff members should help here. However, very often the development and use of a particular guideline or protocol is introduced as part of the pathway and so is part of what you are trying to measure! Again, the thing to do is record your starting point. Was the guideline being applied before the pathway was developed, etc.?
• Environmental changes – these can become particularly important if undertaking some form of before and after study. As various national policy developments diffuse into the NHS they may well impact on the design and focus of the pathway being evaluated. For example the clinical effectiveness initiative, the Calman-Hine report on cancer services (Expert Advisory Group on Cancer, 1995) and more recently the clinical governance initiative (Secretary of State, 1997 p.18) will all arguably have affected the development process and purpose of many ICPs which have been developed in the recent past. It is possible that these initiatives will have altered staff's views concerning multidisciplinary documentation and the use of guidelines, etc. The longer it takes to collect the sample data, the more likely it becomes that this type of confounder will affect the results, leading to the argument that the changes reported are due to other influences and would have happened without the ICP.

Another issue linked with this is how to isolate the pathway from other changes occurring within the organization at the same time. Very often, a number of changes and initiatives are introduced simultaneously as part of a general push to achieve a wider organizational objective. For example, as part of a move to promote clinical effectiveness, there may be structural/managerial changes within the organization, the introduction of new computer systems, and the introduction of guidelines and protocols, new case management systems, etc. Separating these changes from the introduction of the pathway is not easy. Indeed it may be impossible to isolate the pathway as a factor at all. However, this should not stop you undertaking an evaluation. External factors will undoubtedly exert pressure and affect the outcome of the study. What is most important and relevant is to check that the pressures exerted are not out of the ordinary, nor any different from those faced by any NHS organization. If the pressures are unusual or out of the ordinary the transferability and generalizability of the result (i.e. the ability to apply the results to other organizations) is put into question. A study that is undertaken in isolation from the common pressures faced by similar organizations would not make realistic reading in the eyes of another organization that is contemplating developing pathways. In these instances, the best approach is to document the other changes and identify how, if at all, they may have systematically affected the results.

3. Deciding the ICP is operational

If you wish to evaluate the impact of the development of the ICP, think how you will need to decide when the pathway is operational. The literature on pathway development suggests that the development should be quick, perhaps taking as little as three meetings to develop (Overill, 1998). However, this assumes that implementation is successful in all areas, by all those who are responsible for operating it, at the same time. Experience shows that the implementation is rarely as clear-cut as this. Often, some staff may start using the pathway whilst others do not. Different disciplines or staff groups may respond differently, as may staff within different locations. For example, it may be used successfully by all staff in A&E but not used on the in-patient ward. Alternatively, staff may use some aspects of the pathway but not all of them. For example, they may use the pathway documentation but they do not complete the variations. Or they may make the necessary process changes to the clinical care as planned in the pathway but do not record this on the pathway documentation. There are

many different combinations of partial implementation. It is therefore necessary to develop criteria for what you are going to define as successful implementation, so that the evaluation of the impact of the ICP can proceed.

ICPs are intended to be dynamic tools that are regularly reviewed and updated. Particularly at the outset, a pathway will undergo a number of redesigns and alterations based on comments from the staff using it. If the pathway remains the same without alteration for a long period, then it is not operating as a tool for continuous quality improvement and is in danger of stagnating. Again, any measurement of the impact of the pathway needs to take account of this, in order to build into the evaluation the flexibility to allow for these changes and to record them.

Examples of criteria for defining the ICP is operational include:

- agreement of clinical multidisciplinary staff to go 'live' with the ICP;
- completion of ICP documentation by the clinical staff;
- collection of variance data which can be analysed.

4. Use of tools to measure change

The approach chosen to evaluate your ICPs will determine the type of research technique you use to collect the data. Brewer and Hunter (1989, p.17) and McDonald and Daly (1992, p.215) favour an eclectic choice or 'pot pourri' of research techniques combined together, arguing that this will strengthen the reliability of the findings. This employment of multiple methods of investigation – often called 'triangulation' – involves the use of more than one type of data and can combine the collection of quantitative and qualitative research techniques. Proponents of this approach argue that it provides the opportunity to compare and assist in triangulation by bringing different data together and using different methodological viewpoints. ICPs, given their multi-faceted nature, seem to lend themselves to this combination approach.

Reliability

It is important to remember any evaluation tool chosen needs to be reliable. Reliability in practice concerns whether the results from the use of a particular technique can be duplicated if used again and the conditions of the study are unchanged. For example, if you are choosing to observe pathway meetings as part of your evaluation, you may want to consider designing a data collection template. This will make you identify the information you want to collect before the meeting. It will act as a structured reminder as to the precise information you want and will ensure that you do not overlook collecting any of it. It also increases objectivity and helps minimize the risk of bias creeping into the collection of data.

Patient satisfaction

Measuring patient satisfaction is an important aspect of ICP evaluation and one that seems to have been rarely carried out except for a few examples (Falconer et al, 1993; Wright et al., 1997; Stead and Cleary, 1997). Questionnaires, whether completed face-to-face or by post, are the most commonly used form of collecting this information. But this method is not without its problems, as the research literature in this area highlights (McIver, 1991 p.41; Batchelor et al., 1994; Lin and Kelly, 1995; Hall and Dornan, 1988; Locker and Dunt, 1978; Carr-Hill, 1992). There are alternative methods, such as user discussion or focus groups (Ross, 1997 p.42) and critical incident interviews (Flanagan, 1954). The literature recommends using standardized questionnaires (Larsen et al., 1979; McIver, 1991) to ensure reliability and validity, although questionnaires designed specifically in relation to the assessment of ICPs are only just being developed (for example Chou and Boldy, 1999).

Current standardized satisfaction questionnaires tend to address a specific encounter within health services (e.g. one out-patient appointment or one in-patient stay), or to measure the public's views about the NHS overall. Whilst some surveys have been developed to cover a whole condition (e.g. OPCS maternity survey manual, 1989), very few tools appear to be designed to look at users' views of a whole programme of care which may last several months or years for some conditions. Given that one of the fundamental characteristics of an ICP is that it follows the patient through a whole process of care, from start to finish, the need for this type of survey has become essential.

Evaluating ICPs – a way forward

This chapter began by outlining the need for the evaluation of ICPs to answer the question: do ICPs make a difference? One of the complexities of ICPs is that they can include several quality initiatives within the one ICP. For example an ICP may incorporate the latest national guideline for a particular condition; it may also involve the establishment of multi-disciplinary clinical documentation for the first time. In addition the ICP may involve the introduction of new standards of care as well as a change of clinical practice. When evaluating a single ICP it is possible to break down the 'black box' of the tool itself into specific elements or features which are contained within the ICP you are evaluating (de Luc and Currie, 1999). For example if the ICP you are evaluating involves the establishment of multi-disciplinary documentation and the monitoring of outcomes within that new documentation, your evaluation might examine the extent to which communication between the clinical staff has improved along with the legibility and completeness of records. By breaking down the ICP into specific features it allows you to link directly the achievement (or not) of a particular outcome with the consideration of whether a particular feature was present in the ICP.

Alternatively, if you are evaluating a number of ICPs with an organization-wide perspective then it is important to look at the organizational aims identified for the development of the ICPs. For example, are the ICPs being introduced to improve clinical documentation, get evidence into practice and/or as part of a clinical governance strategy. Identifying these organizational aims will assist in identifying the focus of your evaluation.

This chapter has identified the main issues that need to be considered when thinking about undertaking an evaluation of ICPs developed within one's own organization along with suggested approaches for dealing with these complex issues. Figure 9.1 is a checklist of questions one might use when planning an evaluation.

1. What is the purpose of your evaluation (e.g. personal judgement, full research project)?

2. Do you want to evaluate one or more pathways within your organization?

   Single pathway ❏

   Multiple pathways ❏ (how many?)
   _____

3. What outcomes do you want to measure?

   Patient centred ❏

   Clinical staff ❏

   Clinical team ❏

   Organizational ❏

   Other ❏

4. Which type of measurement tool(s) would be most appropriate?

   Experimental ❏

   Survey and/or interview ❏

   Case study ❏

   Participatory action research ❏

5. What baseline information do you need to collect so that you can make a comparison with the care provided when the pathway(s) is operating?
   _____

6. What size sample will suffice for your evaluation?
   _____
   _____

7. Identify the confounders or outside influences which might affect your evaluation.
   Patient characteristics/demographics?
   _____
   _____

   Staff characteristics?
   _____
   _____

   Outside forces/environmental factors?
   _____
   _____

8. List two criteria for defining when your ICP is operational.
   _____
   _____

Figure 9.1 Evaluating ICPs – checklist

References

Bailey, R., Weingarten, S., Lewis, M. and Mohsenifar, Z. (1998) Impact of clinical pathways and practice guidelines on the management of acute exacerbations of bronchial asthma. *Chest*, 113(1), 28–33.

Batchelor, C., Owens, D., Read, M. and Bloor, M. (1994) Patient satisfaction studies: methodology, management and consumer evaluation. *International Journal of Health Care Quality Assurance*, 7(7), 22–30.

Brewer, J. and Hunter, A. (1989) Multimethod research: a synthesis of styles. *Sage Library of Social Research 175*, Sage Publications.

Brown, J. and Simpson, L. (1994) *Co-ordinating patient care: putting principles into practice*. Northallerton Health Services Trust/Department of Health.

Cannon, C., Johnson, B., Cermignani, M., Scirica, B., Sagarin, M. and Walls, R. (1999) Emergency Department Thrombolysis Critical Pathway Reduces Door-to-Drug Times in Acute Myocardial Infarction. *Clinical Cardiology*, 22, 17–20.

Carr-Hill, R. (1992) The measurement of patient satisfaction. *Journal of Public Health Medicine*, 14(3), 236–49.

Chou, S. and Boldy, D. (1999) Patient perceived quality-of-care in hospital in the context of clinical pathways: development of an approach. *Journal of Quality Clinical Practice*, 19(2), 89–93.

Council of International Hospitals (1993a) *The Toronto Hospital: cases a and b*. The Advisory Board, Council of International Hospitals.

Council of International Hospitals (1993b) *Alliant health system: cases a, b and c*. The Advisory Board, Council of International Hospitals.

Currie, L. (1999) Researching Care Pathway Development in the UK. *NT Research*, 4(5), 283–9.

de Luc, K. and Currie, L. (1999) *Developing, Implementing and Evaluating Care Pathways in the UK: The way to go.* Health Services Management Centre Research Report. University of Birmingham.

Del Togno-Armanasco, V., Hopkin, L. and Harter, S. (1993) *Collaborative Nursing Case Management: A Handbook for Development and Implementation.* Springer Publishing Company.

Dowsey, M., Kilgour, M., Santamaria, N. and Choong, P. (1999) Clinical pathways in hip and knee arthroplasty: a prospective randomised controlled study. *Medical Journal of Australia*, 170, 59–62.

Expert Advisory Group on Cancer (1995) *A policy framework for commissioning cancer services.* The Calman-Hine Report. NHS Executive.

Falconer, J., Roth, E., Sutin, J. et al. (1993) The critical path method in stroke rehabilitation: lessons from an experiment in cost containment and outcome improvement. *Quarterly Review Bulletin*, January, 8–16.

Flanagan, J. (1954) The critical incident technique. *Psychological Bulletin*, 51, 327–58.

Gibb, H., Hanson S., Banfield, M. and Doney, G. (1995) *Critical path: an investigation into elderly care in acute hospital settings. Research Report.* Professorial Nursing Unit for Research and Clinical Development, Aged and Extended Care, Southern Sydney Area Health Service, University of Technology, Sydney.

Gibb, H. and Banfield, M. (1996) The issue of critical paths in Australia: where are they taking us? *Nursing Inquiry*, 3, 36–44.

Greengold, N. and Weingarten, S. (1996) Developing evidence-based practice guidelines and pathways. *Journal on Quality Improvement*, 22(6), 391–402.

Hale, C. (1995) Research issues in case management. *Nursing Standard*, 9(44), 29–32.

Hale, C. (1997) Issues in the evaluation of multidisciplinary pathways of care. In Wilson, J. (ed.) *Integrated Care Management: The Path to Success?* Oxford, Butterworth–Heinemann, pp.281–96.

Hall, J. and Dornan, M. (1988) What patients like about their medical care and how often they are asked: a meta-analysis of the satisfaction literature. *Social Science and Medicine*, 27(9), 935–9.

Hofmann, P. (1993) Critical path method: an important tool for co-ordinating clinical care. *Journal on Quality Improvement*, 19(7), 235–46.

Holtzman, J., Bjerke, T. and Kane, R. (1998) The effects of clinical pathways for renal transplant on patient outcomes and length of stay. *Medical Care*, 36(6), 826–34.

Huber, T., Carlton, L., Harward, T. et al. (1998) Impact of a clinical pathway for elective infrarenal aortic reconstructions. *Annals of Surgery*, 227(5), 691–701.

Kwan-Gett, T., Lozano, P., Mullin, K. and Marcuse, E. (1997) One-year experience with an inpatient asthma clinical pathway. *Archives of Paediatric Adolescent Medicine*, 151, 684–9.

Larsen, D., Attkissen, C., Hargreaves, W. and Nguyen, T. (1979) Assessment of client/patient satisfaction: development of a general scale. *Evaluation and Program Planning*, 2, 197–207.

Lewin, K. (1946) Action Research and Minority Problems. *Journal of Social Issues*, 2, 34–6.

Lin, B. and Kelly, E. (1995) Methodological issues in patient satisfaction surveys. *International Journal of Health Care Quality Assurance*, 8(6), 32–7.

Locker, D. and Dunt, D. (1978) Theoretical and methodological issues in sociological studies of consumer satisfaction with medical care. *Social Science and Medicine*, 12(4), 283–92.

McDonald, I. and Daly, J. (1992) Research methods in health care – a summing up. In Daly, J., McDonald, I. and Willis, E. (eds) *Researching Health Care: Designs, Dilemmas, Disciplines.* Routledge, pp.209–16.

McIver, S. (1991) *Obtaining the Views of Outpatients.* King's Fund Centre for Health Services Development.

OPCS (1989) *Women's Experience of the Maternity Care – A Survey Manual.* London, HMSO.

Overill, S. (1998) A practical guide to care pathways. *Journal of Integrated Care*, 2, 93–8.

Parsley, K. (1998) *Exploring the development, implementation and evaluation of patient pathways in Australia.* London, The Florence Nightingale Foundation.

Riley, K. (1998) Paving the way. *Health Service Journal*, 108(5597), 30–31.

Riley, K. (1999) *An evaluation of the contribution packages of care can make to the effectiveness of patient care.* PhD Thesis. Faculty of Commerce and Social Science, University of Birmingham.

Robson, C. (1993) *Real World Research: A Resource for Social Scientists and Practitioner Researchers.* Blackwell.

Ross, L. (1997) Qualitative research methods – data collection and analysis. In Carter, Y. and Thomas, C. (eds) *Research Methods in Primary Care.* Radcliff Medical Press, pp.39–47.

Schriefer, J. (1994) The synergy of pathways and algorithms: two tools work better than one. *Journal on Quality Improvement*, 20(9), 485–99.

Secretary of State for Health (1997) *The new NHS: modern, dependable CM3807.* London, HMSO.

Stead, L. and Cleary, A. (1997) Integrated care pathways within a quality health service. In Wilson, J. (ed.) *Integrated Care Management: The Path to Success?* Oxford, Butterworth–Heinemann, pp.239–61.

Taylor, J. (1997) *Seamless care: examining the role of integrated care pathways.* The Florence Nightingale Foundation/University of Central Lancashire.

Tonges, M. and Brett, J. (1995) Program Evaluation. In Zander, K. (ed.) *Managing Outcomes through Collaborative Care: The Application of Care Mapping and Case Management.* American Hospital Publishing Inc., pp.177–93.

Wright, C., Wain, J. and Grillo, H. et al. (1997) Pulmonary Lobectomy Patient Care Pathway: A Model to Control Cost and Maintain Quality. *Annals of Thoracic Surgery*, 64(2), 299–302.

Clinical benchmarking

Sue Middleton and Adrian Roberts

What is benchmarking?

Benchmarking is essentially about finding and implementing better practice. It involves identifying processes that work elsewhere and if appropriate emulating them. The aim is to reduce duplication by learning from others who have already found the answer(s).

The key to successful benchmarking, however, is 'to know your own organization before seeking to change it'. The starting point of any benchmarking exercise must be a detailed analysis of your own performance. Benchmarking requires a thorough understanding of local processes in order for us to focus on our main problem areas ('failure points') and the action required to achieve change.

> Benchmarking is:
>
> the continuous process of measuring products, services and practices against leaders, allowing the identification of demonstrably better practices which will lead to measurable improvement in performance.
>
> **Or more simply**, 'finding and implementing better practice' (VFM Unit, 1997).

Within the NHS, benchmarking has often been seen as the collection of 'numbers' against a series of defined performance indicators with the results formulated into a 'league table' suggesting comparative levels of performance. Whilst comparative data is *essential* for benchmarking, the danger is that organizations will indulge in data collection with little understanding of the key issues facing the service investigated or the key processes which deliver the performance. The real value of using data within a benchmarking exercise is to highlight areas where attention will lead to better performance, not to provide information on how this better performance may be achieved.

Why is benchmarking important?

Like the question 'do you take regular exercise?' there is only one right answer to 'are you benchmarking?' The agenda faced by all NHS and social care organizations is formidable, with the constant pressures of new guidance, exhortation to higher productivity, increased consumer demand and expectation for new services placing enormous pressure on individuals' time and on organizational integrity.

Benchmarking recognizes that it is impossible for us to find all the answers 'in house' and encourages us to focus our improvement efforts from 'inside out' to take advantage of the lessons we can learn from others. It requires us to visit the department or the organization next door, often resulting in the discovery that different organizations look at the same things in different ways. It also asks us to clarify a vision of the future by defining:

- what we are seeking to achieve (in six months, one year, five years' time);
- where are we starting from (the baseline);
- how will we get there (the action plan).

The concept of learning from the success (and failures) of others is not new but is often undertaken in an ad-hoc manner limiting its potential impact. Benchmarking offers a systematic approach to managing this activity in a way that encourages partnerships between both individuals and organizations.

Performance assessment framework

Recent guidance has emphasized the use of benchmarking to improve performance across the NHS. For example, in order to support local action to increase the priority given to benchmarking, the NHS Executive has undertaken to:

- support the development of the comparative information needed to underpin benchmarking activity;
- encourage the use of comparative information to support the implementation of best practice, by providing easy access to this data on the 'Learning Zone' intranet website;
- identify and publicize beacon providers in the fields of waiting lists and times, primary care, mental health; staff development,

cancer services and health improvement (Department of Health, 1998 pp.22–23).

Similarly, the new Welsh Assembly is committed to developing a national benchmarking programme with the aim of enhancing the quality of care, promoting best practice and achieving best value across the NHS. Trusts will be required to 'benchmark' their major efficiency drivers to strive for improvements in cost, quality and throughput and the programme will see data shared openly with all interested parties in the NHS (NHS Wales, 1998).

Clinical benchmarking

Differences in practice between individual clinicians, and between NHS and social care

Table 10.1 Comparative information available to NHS organizations (Department of Health, 1998 pp.22–23)

Scope of benchmarking	Programmes of care	Trusts	Health authorities
Health improvement	*Assessments for NSF conditions*		Public health common data set HLPIs
Fair access	*Assessment of variation in utilization rates for different conditions relative to need*	*Assessment of variations in admission rates for effective treatments relative to need*	HLPIs Performance tables: various access measures
Effective delivery of appropriate health care	*Assessment of utilization rates for more or less effective treatments for NSF conditions*	*Assessment of admission rates relative to need for more or less effective treatments*	HLPIs Clinical effectiveness indicators
	Effectiveness indicators being developed for specific conditions	Voluntary national audits (e.g. intensive care, National Audit and Research Centre	
Efficiency	*Database of reference costs 'developed to support. . . programmes of care for patients with different needs' (White Paper, para 9.22); in the first instance, for NSF conditions*	Audit Commission Trust Profiles: acute hospital unit costs allowing for casemix and other cost drivers *Investigation of Drivers of Trust efficiency* Schedule of Reference Costs and Reference Cost Index	HLPIs
Patient/carer experience	National Patient Survey (hospitals)	Performance tables: complaints performance; waiting times; *National Patient Survey*	HLPIs Performance tables: waiting times etc National Patient Survey
Health outcomes of NHS care	*Outcome measures being developed for particular diseases*	*Clinical indicators* *Trust level mortality rates for particular procedures*	HLPIs Clinical indicators

Key:
HLPIs = high level performance indicators. *Comparisons under development shown in italics.*

organizations, can result in unnecessary variations in both the quality of care and patient outcomes. Clinical benchmarking, the direct comparison of clinical practice and service delivery, provides the means to:

- compare the inputs and results of both clinical practice and service delivery;
- ensure that outcomes are the results of processes;
- support clinical effectiveness initiatives incorporating evidence-based medicine;
- complete the clinical audit cycle;
- solve problems of patient flow and inappropriate bed management.

Benchmarking can also be used together with ICPs to:

- test the existing clinical process in terms of evidence and good practice before it is formalized into a pathway – there is little point in writing a pathway based on poor practice;
- improve existing clinical pathways during review and evaluation.

Critical success factors

The process of benchmarking is relatively simple but it takes application to be successful. In particular it is imperative to spend time on communication and building commitment. There are a number of critical success factors that need to be in place within an organization for their benchmarking to be successful. These can be defined as:

- a commitment to continuous improvement;
- sponsorship at senior level;
- a willingness to understand how your organization works before seeking to change it;
- a willingness to learn from others;
- good internal communication;
- good project management and the ability to form the right team;
- a tradition of seeing initiatives through to completion.

The stages of benchmarking: the 12-step benchmarking plan

The NHS Benchmarking Reference Centre, established in 1992, has developed a 12-step plan for initiating and managing benchmarking projects. This plan is fully documented in the 'benchmarking workbook' (Bullivant, 1997). A tried and tested methodology, it is based on good communication and project management skills and follows a logical process: getting started, collecting and analysing information and managing and reviewing the process of change. Experience shows that attempts to short-circuit it can often prolong the benchmarking project rather than shorten it.

Table 10.2 outlines the key activities in the 12-step benchmarking plan.

Getting started

In practice, the time spent on 'getting started' ensures that your benchmarking project is worthwhile, is focused on failure points within the process and has the necessary commitment to proceed. Getting started can be synthesized into the following steps (see also Figure 10.1):

1. Define the desired outcome(s) of the activity under investigation.
2. Define and set the start point of the activity.
3. Agree the boundaries and identify related issues and departments but do not map or tackle them for the moment.
4. Identify and map the 6–10 high-level process elements that you use now to deliver the service objective.
5. Identify failure points and responsibilities; decide if failure points can be corrected, require search for better practice or more detailed mapping of process or performance. Only investigate the impact of related departments if they are part of the failure point.
6. Use the above to define the project, data requirements and likely benchmarking partners.

At this stage of 'getting started' the project team will have a completed set of process maps and have identified a number of failure points and opportunities for improvement. The 'getting started' phase of developing an ICP is used to produce the same products (i.e. process maps, failure points, opportunities for improvement). In this context, the development of ICPs can be seen as a logical way of initiating a benchmarking exercise.

Table 10.3 outlines the similarities between the getting started phases of ICPs and benchmarking.

Table 10.2 The 12-step benchmarking plan

Benchmarking stages	*Key activities*
Benchmarking: getting started	
1. Identify key issue to benchmark	• Identify appropriate project
2. Define SMART stretch goals and the process to benchmark	• Define the future outcomes you wish to achieve • Draw high level process map(s)
3. Identify information required	• Identify problem areas ('failure points'), opportunities for improvement and data requirements • Undertake more detailed process mapping if required
4. Identify who needs to be involved	• Select members of the benchmarking team • Identify any external support required • Gain appropriate approval to continue
Benchmarking: information and analysis	
5. Collect the information, select and contact benchmarking partners	• Define your benchmarking project using the information collated during 'getting started' • Identify and contact potential benchmarking partners
6. Determine and verify the gap in performance	• Analyse your own data against your chosen partner(s) • Undertake benchmarking visit if appropriate
7. Establish difference in process	• Compare current practice • Undertake benchmarking visit if appropriate
8. Target future performance	• Develop an action plan to achieve change
Benchmarking change: project management	
9. Communication and commitment	• Communicate to all staff involved how findings have been reached and the reasons behind any change(s)
10. Establishing the change team	• Select any new members required to make the agreed change(s)
11. Implementation	• Recognize responsibility to produce a defined result by an agreed date, with the necessary actions broken down into clear, manageable steps
12. Review progress and recalibrate	• Review progress against defined outcomes (Step 2) and identify what could be done better next time • If necessary, return to Step 1

Table 10.3 Getting started – clinical pathways and benchmarking

Getting started: integrated clinical pathways	*Getting started: benchmarking*
1. Select appropriate client group	1. Identify key issue to benchmark
2. Agree scope of the pathway: start-point, end-point and boundaries	2. Define the desired outcome
3. Choose the development team	3. Agree the boundaries and identify related issue
4. Define the desired outcome(s) of care	4 Map the current process.
5. Map the current process of care	5. Identify failure points, measuring points and responsibilities
6. Evaluate current practice, identifying any failure points and/or opportunities for improvement	6 Choose the benchmarking team.
Outcome: Development team, process maps, failure points and opportunities for improvement	**Outcome**: Benchmarking team, process maps, failure points and opportunities for improvement

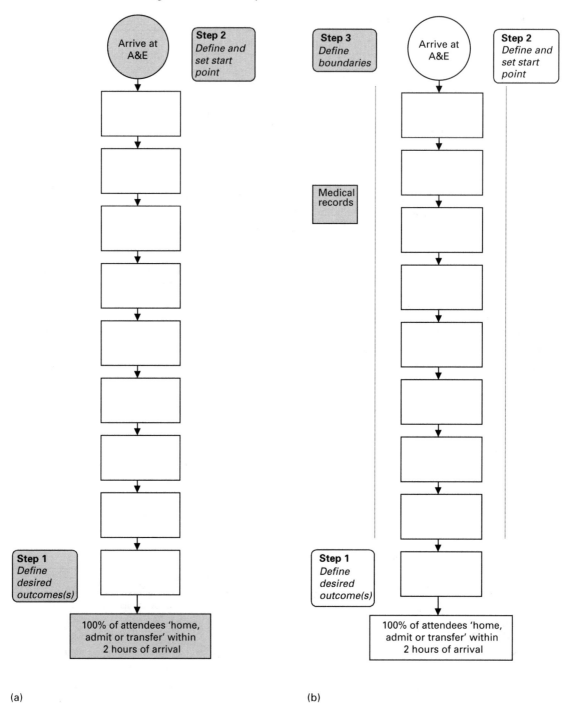

(a)　　　　　　　　　　　　　　　　　　　　(b)

Figure 10.1 Benchmarking: getting started (an example)

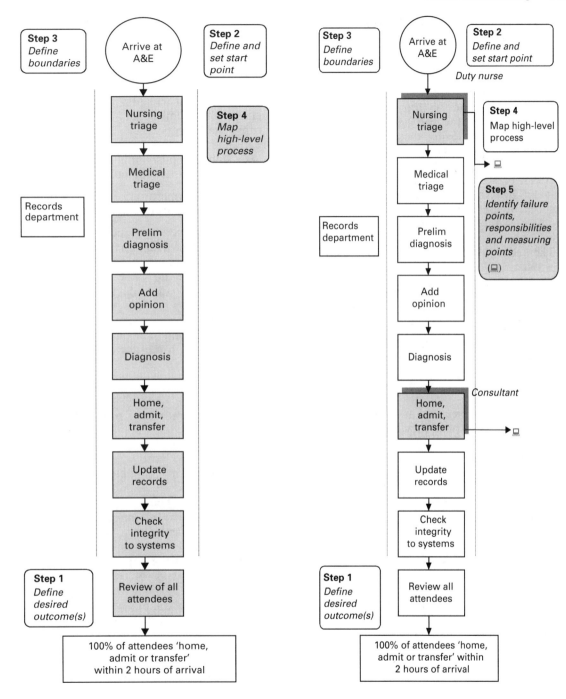

Step 3 *Define boundaries*

Step 2 *Define and set start point*

Arrive at A&E

Step 4 *Map high-level process*

Nursing triage

Medical triage

Records department

Prelim diagnosis

Add opinion

Diagnosis

Home, admit, transfer

Update records

Check integrity to systems

Step 1 *Define desired outcome(s)*

Review of all attendees

100% of attendees 'home, admit or transfer' within 2 hours of arrival

(c)

Step 3 *Define boundaries*

Step 2 *Define and set start point*

Arrive at A&E

Duty nurse

Nursing triage

Step 4 Map high-level process

Medical triage

Step 5 *Identify failure points, responsibilities and measuring points*

Records department

Prelim diagnosis

Add opinion

Diagnosis

Consultant

Home, admit, transfer

Update records

Check integrity to systems

Step 1 *Define desired outcome(s)*

Review all attendees

100% of attendees 'home, admit or transfer' within 2 hours of arrival

(d)

Figure 10.1 (continued) Benchmarking: getting started (an example)

Analysing current performance and opportunities for improvement

This stage of benchmarking is essentially an assessment of *current* performance against the desired outcomes defined for the activity under investigation. A step or activity that 'adds value' to the process is one that contributes to achieving these outcomes. By examining the process maps it may be possible to identify areas of inefficiency or duplication that can be solved in a fairly straightforward manner (by removing one of the process steps, for example). However, more complex problems will require more detailed investigation.

The key is to consider all possible causes for a problem by looking at the entire process. It is also important for the benchmarking team to be prepared to challenge existing beliefs and to avoid the temptation to focus on solutions rather than the problem itself. For example, delays in getting patients to theatre on time may be explained 'by not enough porters'. However, the real problem is the delay, not the assumed reason of 'porters'.

It is also important to remember that problems are often caused at a different point in the process to where they *appear*. Without a correct assessment of the failure points within the system, it is unlikely that the solutions will have the required impact on performance. With this in mind, the benchmarking team will also need to collect some data to validate the problem area (i.e. these figures confirm to us that this is the problem) and to use as a basis for comparison.

In order to highlight the real failure points in the process, it may be necessary to undertake some more detailed process mapping. Guidance on more detailed mapping can be found in **Chapter 5, Getting started**. Begin by mapping potential failure points in more detail as it is unlikely the same level of detail will be required for elements of the process that are working well.

Opportunities for improvement

When assessing opportunities for improvement, experience has shown that a number of common themes can be identified. It is particularly important to remember that 'failures' tend to occur at the points in the process where responsibility is passed from one member of staff to another or between different departments. It is therefore worth investigating the potential to:

- ensure the start point of the process is the same for all participants;
- reduce the number of 'hand-off' points within the process;
- rearrange tasks so that they can be undertaken simultaneously or in to an order more suitable for all participants.

In addition, in terms of establishing a patient focus, it is important to assess whether:

- services can be provided closer to the patient (e.g. moving services from acute care to the community);
- process steps of no value can be removed (e.g. recording patient details on more than one occasion);
- customized processes can be defined for patients with common characteristics (e.g. different access routes for elective and non-elective patients).

Finding benchmarking partners

At this stage of benchmarking, the project team will have produced what is essentially a baseline review. The completed process maps, defined failure points and opportunities for improvement can be shared with better performers with the intention of identifying areas of good practice that can be incorporated or adapted locally. However, identifying appropriate benchmarking partners is not always easy if the data you require to establish a 'performance gap' is not routinely published or is not available in a meaningful form.

This is not so much of a problem if the impetus for your benchmarking project is derived from a poor set of results against a 'league table' of indicators – you can simply approach the members of the data set who are classed as high performers. Similarly, if you are conducting an internal benchmarking exercise on specific clinical conditions, partners can be drawn from within your own organization.

If these options are unavailable, there are a number of other techniques you can use to help identify benchmarking partners. These include searching the literature around your subject (and in addition to professional journals you may wish to consider conference speakers, newspapers, annual reports and directories of good practice) and using existing professional networks (e.g. professional associations, benchmarking clubs, local networks). Alternatively, it may be worth approaching a number of organizations that you feel may have an interest in the area of activity under investigation. In this case, the means of performance comparison can be defined and agreed between the participants.

Using maturity matrices

For areas that are difficult to compare in terms of numbers, or for a full comparison of 'qualitative' issues, it may be appropriate to consider using a benchmarking tool called a maturity matrix. Maturity matrices are designed to enable organizations to assess their current performance and to set goals for future improvements. They present the essential elements of a chosen issue, performance measures (where valid), a number of critical success factors and a performance grid, indicating for each element of the issue the minimum standard and good and better practice levels.

For internal purposes, maturity matrices can provide an excellent framework for departmental meetings to help define current performance and what action can be taken to improve. They also allow comparisons with performers who are achieving better practice. Because they are simple to use and understand, they can be sent to organizations believed to be performing well, inviting them to compare practice and performance, concentrating on areas recognized as needing improvement.

An example of a maturity matrix focusing on the development and implementation of ICPs is presented in Appendix 1.

Choice of benchmarking partner

Ultimately, the *choice* of benchmarking partner(s) will depend on two factors, namely

- validation of the information used to establish the performance gap (i.e. you will want to confirm that you are working with a better performer)

- the relationship between the organizations involved (i.e. is it or will it be a good one, are they prepared to cooperate).

Benchmarking visits

Benchmarking visits can be an effective means of cementing relationships between benchmarking partners. They are, however, a means to an end – improved performance. Visits should be conducted in line with the protocol (see box), which is adapted from the Benchmarking Code of Conduct (VFM Unit, 1998).

Protocol for benchmarking visits

- Provide an agenda in advance.
- Be professional, honest, courteous and prompt.
- Introduce all attendees and explain why they are present.
- Keep to the agenda.
- Use language that is universal, not jargon.
- Be sure that neither partner is disclosing proprietary information unless both parties (with the proper authority) have obtained prior approval.
- Share information about your own process and from study results.
- Offer to facilitate a future reciprocal visit.
- Conclude meetings and visits on schedule.
- Thank your benchmarking partner for their time and for sharing their process.

If the visit is successful, it will often indicate opportunities for both partners to improve performance. This is the main reason that benchmarking remains attractive to better performers. In addition, it is worth sharing results and arranging reciprocal visits focusing on other areas of potential investigation.

Learning from others

Sharing your processes and data with your chosen partner(s) will give you plenty of material to undertake a critical comparison of process which will help you to explain the 'performance gap'. It is important at this stage to be organizationally honest and not to seek to explain away differences in performance with excuses but, on the other hand, it is also necessary not to take all the information you have collected at face value. You should work through the differences in process with your partner(s) and analyse them within their context. This will give you a better idea of which areas of good practice it is appropriate for you to emulate or to adapt to suit your local environment. An effective way of doing this is to draw an 'improved' process map, identifying the changes involved and the resources (money, training, etc.) required to implement them.

The action plan

Implementing identified changes in practice will require a detailed action plan and a sound project management approach. This will include agreement to produce the defined changes within an agreed timescale, with all actions detailed in a step-by-step project plan. In the first instance the changes should be implemented in 'pilot' form only, with all the staff involved ensured that they will only become permanent if success can be demonstrated against a set of pre-determined criteria. Relationships should be maintained with existing benchmarking partners throughout this period – they might well have been through the same changes and can offer you the benefits of the lessons they will have learned.

Conclusions

It has been a common feature within the NHS for organizations and individuals to take a cautious view of benchmarking, with concerns expressed that failure to comply with a set of externally set targets or 'benchmarks' may lead to adverse publicity or other penalties against participants. However, in its true form, benchmarking is not about compliance but about achievement and the opportunity to improve. Providing we can establish our baseline position and define what we wish to achieve, then benchmarking offers us the structure to discover and make the necessary change to 'bridge the gap'. True, benchmarking is not a universal solution to all the problems we face and it is not an appropriate technique to use in every situation. It can be time consuming and demands commitment to succeed but it is also worth the effort it requires. When internal improvement programmes can not tackle the problems we need to solve, benchmarking offers us the co-ordinated framework to take advantage of innovation and good practice from elsewhere – from within the NHS, the rest of the public sector and beyond.

Benchmarking vision

- Move away from compliance to achievement.
- No surveys or visits without review of goals, process and focus for improvement.
- Look-alike groups are a means to an end, use them but look elsewhere too.
- Promote success.

References

Bullivant, John (1997) *Introduction to benchmarking for continuous improvement in health and local government: workbook*. Wrexham, Benchmarking Reference Centre.

Department of Health (1998) *The NHS Performance Assessment Framework*. Leeds, NHS Executive.

NHS Wales (1998) *Putting Patients First*. Cardiff, Welsh Office.

VFM Unit (1997) *Introduction to benchmarking*. Wrexham, Benchmarking Reference Centre.

VFM Unit (1998) *Benchmarking Visits*. Wrexham, Benchmarking Reference Centre.

Appendices

Appendix 1
Clinical pathways maturity matrix

GOOD PRACTICE MATURITY MATRIX

Clinical pathways: development & implementation

GOOD PRACTICE MATURITY MATRICES

Good practice maturity matrices are designed to enable organizations to assess their current performance in comparison with others and to set goals for future improvements. All organizations should at least be achieving the minimum standards described overleaf and should aspire to the better practice level. However, organizations should also aim to achieve a balance in performance. It is usually better to consolidate all elements at the good practice level rather than to excel at some features and fail in others.

Good practice maturity matrices focus on organizational key issues as recommended in the European Foundation for Quality Management (EFQM) framework.

INTRODUCTION TO THE TOPIC

Clinical pathways are both a case management and a clinical audit tool. They allow a multidisciplinary team to coordinate care by setting out all the activities involved in the care of a patient with a defined condition. They lead each patient towards a set of desired outcomes and ensure that specified interventions are delivered at the right time, by the right professional in the right way.

In essence, the pathway provides a multidisciplinary plan of care and by following this plan unnecessary variations in practice and outcomes among patients within the same diagnosis can be reduced. It is a guide to usual treatment patterns and does not compromise the need for clinical judgement.

The development of clinical pathways should be seen within the context of significant changes within the NHS. They are one response to the need for providers to restructure care to ensure effectiveness and efficiency without compromising quality.

TARGET AUDIENCE:

Management executive/team, clinical pathways coordinators, clinical staff, patient interest groups

KEY ACTIVITES

1. Organizational strategy
2. Leadership
3. Commissioner involvement
4. Education
5. Ownership
6. Professional relationships
7. Managing expectations
8. Support
9. Clinical effectiveness
10. Implementation
11. Analysis

CRITICAL SUCCESS FACTORS

1. Pathways are included as part of the organizational quality programme.
2. Collaboration exists between professional groups with a strong medical lead.
3. Pathways are based on evidence and best practice and include an objective, goals and outcomes.
4. Project facilitators have appropriate skills and the expectations of staff are carefully managed.
5. Variations from the pathway are collated and analysed and used to change clinical practice if appropriate.
6. There is a rolling education programme with appropriate support.
7. Pathways are 'owned' by clinical staff and are completed by all staff involved.

ACTIVITIES	MINIMUM PRACTICE	GOOD PRACTICE	BETTER PRACTICE
Organizational strategy	Decision taken to develop pathways at directorate level.	Decision taken to develop pathways on an organizational basis.	Pathways integrated as part of organizational continuous quality improvement strategy.
Leadership	Senior clinical staff supportive of pathways identified.	Initial pathway development focused on areas with support of senior clinical staff.	Lead for the development of pathways provided by senior clinical staff.
Commissioner involvement	Commissioners aware of development of pathways by local providers.	Local commissioners active in encouraging the development of clinical pathways.	Evidence that commissioning is based upon patient outcomes and clinical pathways.
Education	Training needs of appropriate staff assessed.	Members of pathway development teams trained to provide on-going support to their peers throughout implementation stage.	A rolling programme of education and support, based on needs assessment, is established.
Ownership	Initial pathway development focused on areas where staff are enthusiastic.	Pathway development teams include a representative from each of the professions and/or agencies who provide care and support for chosen group of patients.	Pathways 'owned' by all clinical staff.
Professional relationships	Forum available for multidisciplinary debate.	Pathways developed through multidisciplinary debate.	Evidence available of full collaboration between professional groups.
Managing expectations	Expectations of all appropriate staff are assessed.	Awareness and education programmes developed to remove misconceptions.	Project managers are fully aware of staff expectations which are managed accordingly.
Support	Facilitator appointed to guide pathway development and facilitate collaboration between professional groups.	Full needs assessment of skills required by project manager undertaken.	Project managers fully trained with appropriate facilitation, audit and change management skills.
Clinical effectiveness	Local policy on clinical effectiveness in place.	Pathways based on available evidence or 'best practice' and contain outcomes.	(1) Pathways revised accordingly as new evidence appears. (2) Pathways used to address national initiatives.
Implementation	Appropriate topic chosen for pathway development.	(1) Current practice is recorded and shared. (2) Pathway written by multidisciplinary development team.	Pathways are completed by all appropriate staff – opportunity for regular feedback is established.
Analysis	Variations from pathways are recorded.	Variations from pathways are recorded and collated.	Variations from pathways and outcomes are analysed and used to support changes in practice.

Appendix 2

Integrated care pathway for 'cardiac' chest pain/suspected myocardial infarction

Kidderminster Health Care NHS Trust

Part 1

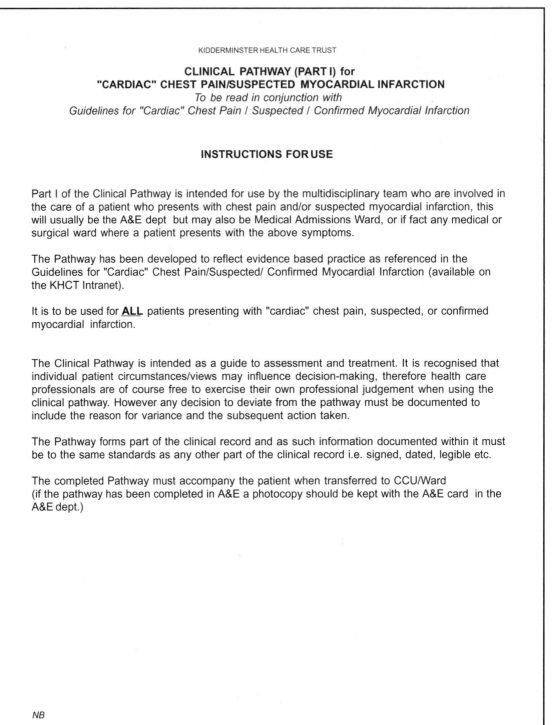

KIDDERMINSTER HEALTH CARE TRUST

CLINICAL PATHWAY (PART I) for
"CARDIAC" CHEST PAIN/SUSPECTED MYOCARDIAL INFARCTION
To be read in conjunction with
Guidelines for "Cardiac" Chest Pain / Suspected / Confirmed Myocardial Infarction

INSTRUCTIONS FOR USE

Part I of the Clinical Pathway is intended for use by the multidisciplinary team who are involved in the care of a patient who presents with chest pain and/or suspected myocardial infarction, this will usually be the A&E dept but may also be Medical Admissions Ward, or if fact any medical or surgical ward where a patient presents with the above symptoms.

The Pathway has been developed to reflect evidence based practice as referenced in the Guidelines for "Cardiac" Chest Pain/Suspected/ Confirmed Myocardial Infarction (available on the KHCT Intranet).

It is to be used for **ALL** patients presenting with "cardiac" chest pain, suspected, or confirmed myocardial infarction.

The Clinical Pathway is intended as a guide to assessment and treatment. It is recognised that individual patient circumstances/views may influence decision-making, therefore health care professionals are of course free to exercise their own professional judgement when using the clinical pathway. However any decision to deviate from the pathway must be documented to include the reason for variance and the subsequent action taken.

The Pathway forms part of the clinical record and as such information documented within it must be to the same standards as any other part of the clinical record i.e. signed, dated, legible etc.

The completed Pathway must accompany the patient when transferred to CCU/Ward
(if the pathway has been completed in A&E a photocopy should be kept with the A&E card in the A&E dept.)

NB
Please do not file this page in patient notes i.e. detach from pathway and destroy

Version 4   KIDDERMINSTER HEALTH CARE TRUST
                              CLINICAL PATHWAY (Part I)
                "CARDIAC" CHEST PAIN / SUSPECTED MYOCARDIAL INFARCTION
                            To be read in conjunction with
              Guidelines for "Cardiac" Chest Pain / Suspected or Confirmed Myocardial Infarction
                              (Please see instructions for use)

Name: _____   A&E No: _____

DOOR (*Nurse to complete this section*)

- **12 lead ECG recorded** (*within 5 minutes of arrival*) ❑
- RMO fast bleeped ❑
- Continuous cardiac monitoring in progress ❑
- Oxygen 100% commenced ❑
- Vital signs recorded at least every 15 minutes

| 200 |
| 190 |
| 180 |
| 170 |
| 160 |
| 150 |
| 140 |
| 130 |
| 120 |
| 110 |
| 100 |
| 90 |
| 80 |
| 70 |
| 60 |
| 50 |
| 40 |
| 30 |
| 20 |

If there are any variances to pathway please give reason and action taken

DATA   (*Dr to complete this section*)

- **(A) Indications for thrombolysis**

  - Central crushing chest pain for 15 minutes not
    relieved by oxygen rest or GTN spray.   Yes / No
  - Time of onset within 12 hours   Yes / No
  - Confirmation from RMO that ECG shows
    evidence of Acute Myocardial Infarction   Yes / No

- **(B) Contra indications to immediate thrombolysis in   A&E**

  - Aortic Dissection - sudden onset extreme tearing
    type chest pain radiating to back and loss of
    peripheral pulses.   Yes / No
  - Known bleeding diathesis (bleeding tendency)   Yes / No
  - CVA, GI bleed, within 3 months   Yes / No
  - Uncontrolled severe hypertension
    (diastolic BP>110 / systolic BP>190)   Yes / No
  - Surgery or long bone trauma within past 6 weeks Yes / No
  - Prolonged traumatic CPR (> 15 minutes
    +/- rib #, >one attempt at central line etc.) Yes / No
  - Current pregnancy   Yes / No
  - Previous thrombolytic agent   Yes / No
  - Age under 30 years   Yes / No

Time of onset of patient symptoms [   ]   **Time patient called for help** [   ]

Time of patients arrival in A&E [   ]   **Time patient commenced thrombolysis** [   ]

D3 DECISION (*Dr to complete this section*)(* delete as appropriate)

* ECG is equivocal
 Provisional diagnosis ....

* ECG shows evidence of acute myocardial infarction
 i.e. ST elevation > 1-2 mm or LBBB thought to be new

- There are clear indications for thrombolysis
 i.e. all answers to part (A) overleaf are yes ☐

- There are <u>NO</u> identified Contra indications
 i.e. all answers to part (B) overleaf are no ☐
 (*if yes to any of (B) seek advice from senior medical officer*)

- **PATIENT TO RECEIVE THROMBOLYSIS IN A&E *YES /*NO**
 (This decision must only be made by RMO or Consultant)

D4 DRUG - Prescriptions/Administration
 (delete as appropriate)

- Oral ASPIRIN 300 mgs Sig......................... Time............
- GTN SPRAY 400mcg x 2 Sig......................... Time............
 repeat as required
- I.V. DIAMORPHINE 5mg Sig......................... Time............
 (mix 5mgs/5mls saline and give increments of 1mg per minute.)
- I.V. METOCLOPROMIDE 10 mgs Sig....................................
 (with first dose of Diamorphine)
- **Signature of Dr prescribing** ....

 If Decision has been made to Thrombolyse :- ....

- Obtain verbal consent for thrombolysis ☐

Give :

I.V. STREPTOKINASE 1.5 MEGAUNITS OVER 60 MINUTES

Signature of Dr prescribing ....

Signature of person administering ....

Time Infusion commenced ....

TRANSFER (*Nurse transferring patient to complete this section*)

- Ensure patient / relatives aware of transfer details ☐
- Porter fast bleeped to transfer patient to CCU .... (Time)
- Patient / Relatives aware of transfer details ☐
- This form, ECG, and photocopy of A&E card sent with patient ☐
- Equipment / personnel for safe transfer available: ☐
 (*Monitor / Defibrillator / Cardiac Drugs / Pocket Mask
 Oxygen & suction / Dr to escort*)
- **Time left department** ....
- Bloods taken in A&E   Yes / No
 (*if Potassium required urgently this can be done in CCU*)

 TRANSFERRED TO: CCU MAW OTHER ....

If there are any variances to Pathway please give reason and action taken

---

NAME (BLOCK CAPITALS) AND SIGNATURE

A&E NURSE.. A&E DR ....

RMO .... TRANSFERRING NURSE ....

Part 2

CLINICAL PATHWAY (PART II) for
"CARDIAC" CHEST PAIN / SUSPECTED / CONFIRMED MYOCARDIAL INFARCTION

(To be read in conjunction with Guidelines for "Cardiac" Chest Pain/Suspected/ Confirmed Myocardial Infarction

INSTRUCTIONS FOR USE

Part II of the Clinical Pathway is intended for use by the multidisciplinary team who are involved in the care of a patient with "cardiac" chest pain, suspected and/or confirmed acute myocardial infarction, from admission to CCU through to discharge. NB Part I of the pathway should already have been completed in the area (usually A&E) where the patient first presented.

The Pathway has been developed to reflect evidence-based practice as referenced in the Guidelines for "Cardiac" Chest Pain/Suspected/ Confirmed Myocardial Infarction (available on the KHCT Intranet).

It is to be used for ALL patients presenting with "cardiac" chest pain, suspected, or confirmed Myocardial Infarction.

The Clinical Pathway is intended as a guide to assessment and treatment. It is recognized that individual patient circumstances/views may influence decision-making, therefore health care professionals are of course free to exercise their own professional judgement when using the care pathway. However any decision to deviate from the pathway must be documented (in the UPR) to include the reason for variance and the subsequent action taken.

The Pathway forms part of the clinical record and as such information documented within it must be to the same standards as any other part of the clinical record i.e. signed, dated, legible etc.

The Clinical Pathway should be used in conjunction with and inserted into the Unified Patient Record

- Interventions:
  The interventions should be signed off as completed. Some interventions may be relevant for all nursing shifts e.g. 'BP and HR recorded 4 hourly' however some such as 'cannula removed' can obviously only be carried out once! If so please enter N/A in box.
  If an intervention is amended/not carried out for any other reason please enter "V" (variance) in box and document this variance from the pathway in the UPR with details of the reason for variance and the subsequent action taken.

- Goals:
  Any goals NOT met should be marked with a V (variance) and detailed in the UPR, including information explaining reasons and action to be taken.

- Outcomes:
  The Outcome Form must be completed as indicated in pathway. Information collected will be used to amend pathway/guidelines and/or address highlighted issues in order to ensure that clinically effective care is continually provided.

If you have any comments and / or any query or difficulties completing the pathway, please contact:
Sally Davis (Specialist Nurse - CHD) ext. 3307

ABBREVIATIONS **USED IN PATHWAY:**

A&E	Accident and Emergency	COAD	Chronic Obstructive Airways Disease	HR	Heart Rate
AMI	Acute Myocardial Infarction	COPD	Chronic Obstructive Pulmonary Disease	IU	International Unit
AST	Aspartase Transaminase	CPR	Cardio Pulmonary Resuscitation	IV	Intravenous
BP	Blood Pressure	D/N	District Nurse	L	Late Shift
CCU	Coronary Care Unit	E	Early Shift	LBBB	Left Bundle Branch Block
C&E	Creatinine and Electrolytes	ECG	Electrocardiogram	LV	Left Ventricular
CK	Creatine Kinase	FBC	Full Blood Count	N	Night Shift
CNS	Clinical Nurse Specialist	GI	Gastrointestinal	UPR	Unified Patient Record
RMO	Resident Medical Officer	GTN	Glyceryl Trinitrate		

NB Please do not file this page in patient notes i.e. detach from pathway and destroy

CLINICAL PATHWAY (PART II) for
"CARDIAC" CHEST PAIN / SUSPECTED or CONFIRMED MYOCARDIAL INFARCTION
To be read in conjunction with the
Guidelines for "Cardiac" Chest Pain/Suspected or Confirmed Myocardial Infarction
(Please see instructions for use and ensure your full signature is recorded at the end of the pathway)

NAME... Unit No...................................

STAGE 1 ADMISSION Date......./...../....... TIME OF ADMISSION TO CCU................
If patient has had an equivocal ECG (i.e. AMI not yet confirmed)   please complete **Section 1a**
If patient has confirmed AMI and <u>has</u> received thrombolysis in A&E   please complete **Section 1b**

SECTION 1a EQUIVOCAL ECG

Nursing interventions:	
• ECG repeated at 30, 60 and 120 minutes or immediately if in pain	**Signature**
• For advice or confirmation re ECG change contact ITU via fax: 01562 513011	
• Continuous cardiac monitoring - MCL1 hook up	
• Continuous oxygen 100% (24% if COAD present)	....
• BP and HR recorded at least every 15 minutes	

Medical interventions

• Diamorphine / Metaclopramide/Nitrates prescribed on "p r n" basis

• Obtain enzyme results and discuss thrombolysis with consultant if appropriate

• Check history for indications / contraindications for thrombolysis: *(Circle Yes/No as appropriate)*

Indications for thrombolysis	
• Central crushing chest pain for 15 minutes not relieved by oxygen, rest or GTN spray	Yes / No
• Time of onset of symptoms within 12 hours (**TIME OF ONSET** ....)	Yes / No
• ECG showing evidence of Acute Myocardial Infarction	Yes / No
Contraindications to Thrombolysis	
• Aortic Dissection (sudden onset extreme tearing type chest pain radiating to back and loss of peripheral pulses.	Yes / No
• Known bleeding diathesis (bleeding tendency)	Yes / No
• Significant risk of potential hemorrhage e.g. previous sub-arachnoid hemorrhage <u>ever</u> or cerebral or GI bleed, within past 3 months	Yes / No
• Uncontrolled severe hypertension(diastolic>1 10:systolic>1 90)	Yes / No
• Surgery or long bone trauma within past 6 weeks	Yes / No
• Prolonged traumatic CPR (>15 min +/- rib **#**, >one attempt at central line etc.)	Yes / No
• Current pregnancy	Yes / No
• Age under 30 years	Yes / No

- 1 -

NAME.. Unit No...................................

Decision: Patient to receive thrombolysis   Yes ☐   No[1] ☐

         If so which type[2]   Streptokinase ☐   Reteplase ☐

- Verbal consent obtained for thrombolysis ☐
- Prescribe oral Metoprotol
- If Reteplase is prescribed, also prescribe heparin IV prior to, and following Reteplase therapy[3]

Dr's signature...

SECTION 1b CARE DURING ADMINISTRATION OF THROMBOLYSIS

TIME INFUSION GIVEN / COMMENCED ....

Nursing interventions:

- Patient to be kept on bed rest
- BP and HR recorded every 15 minutes
- Continuous cardiac monitoring
- ECG repeated within 1 hour of commencement of thrombolytic therapy
- Monitor for adverse side effects to thrombolysis

Signature

....

SECTION 1c CONTINUATION OF CARE FOR 1ST 24 HOURS

Nursing interventions:	E	L	N
• BP and HR recorded 4 hourly			
• Oxygen saturation recorded 4 hourly			
• Puncture / cannula sites checked 4 hourly			
• Waterlow score recorded in UPR, including action to be taken if considered 'at risk'			
• Explanation given to patient re pressure area care			
• Explanation given to patient re 'what a heart attack is' / importance of reporting any pain / equipment / procedures etc			
• Family informed of diagnosis / progress / visiting times (*see 'patient wishes on releasing confidential information' on UPR*)			
• Mobility programme explained to patient **before they leave CCU**			

[1] If a diagnosis other than acute MI is made (e.g. unstable angina) please exit pathway and return to normal documentation. If a diagnosis of AMI is made but thrombolysis is inappropriate, please document reasons in UPR and continue to Section 1c of pathway.

[2] If streptokinase has ever been administered more than 4 days previously it should not be given again and reteplase should be given as an alternative. Reteplase should also be given to any patient under the age of 50 with a large anterior infarct.

[3] Heparin should be administered concomitantly with and following the administration of reteplase to reduce the risk of re-thrombolysis. The recommended heparin dose is 5000 I.U. given as a bolus intravenous injection prior to reteplase therapy followed by an infusion of 1000 I.U. per hour starting after the second reteplase bolus. Heparin should be administered for at least 24 hours, preferably for 48 (-72) hours, aiming to keep aPTT values 1.5 to 2 times normal.

NAME... Unit No...................................

GOALS: *If not met please document details in UPR*	E	L	N
I. Pain / nausea adequately controlled			
II. Patient able to meet hygiene needs with moderate assistance			
III. Bed / chair rest			
IV. Tolerating acceptable level of diet and oral fluids			
V. Anxiety level within acceptable limits			

Medical interventions:	Dr's signature
• Initial blood samples for C&E's / FBC / CK and AST levels / Glucose / Cholesterol taken and sent to lab on admission *(check not already obtained and sent from A&E)* **NB Please mark urgent and record date and <u>time</u> blood obtained on form**	
• Repeat CK/AST levels 10-12 hrs after admission **(only if initial levels were normal)** **NB Please record date and <u>time</u> blood obtained on form**	
• Chest x-ray booked Departmental ☐ Portable ☐ *(must be performed within 24 hrs of admission to CCU)*	
• Prescribe prophylactic subcutaneous heparin following **Streptokinase**	
• Prescribe Ace Inhibitors if patient shows evidence of LV dysfunction *(to be commenced 24 hours after AMI)*	
• Prescribe 75 mgs oral aspirin daily (unless contraindicated)	
• If blood glucose is over 10 mmols/litre commence insulin sliding scale for 24 hours and if actually diabetic consider maintaining on insulin long term	

Multidisciplinary notes for 1st 24 hours	Sig/designation

OUTCOMES
Prior to patient leaving CCU please complete Section A on outcome form at the back of the Pathway

NAME.. Unit No....................................

TRANSFER TO MEDICAL WARD [4] Date......./...../....... Time.....................			
Nursing interventions: (Prior to or immediately following transfer)	**E**	**L**	**N**
• Patient and relatives informed of transfer			
• Menu diverted			
• Thrombolytic card attached to pathway			
• Patients own medication sent home and drugs ordered from pharmacy as necessary			
• CNS-HD informed of admission bleep 3307 (or *leave message on answer-phone*)			
• ECG Dept informed of admission - bleep 3355 *(if weekend inform Monday)*			
STAGE 2 [5] Date commenced Stage 2 care ..../...../.......			
Nursing interventions:	**E**	**L**	**N**
• Cannula removed - site checked			
• Chest stickers removed			
• Record BP and HR 4 hourly			
• Episodes of pain assessed and documented in UPR (type *I* severity *I* duration / location)			
• Explanation of Mobility Programme reinforced			
• 'Recovery from Heart Disease' Booklet given			
GOALS: *If not met please document details in UPR*	**E**	**L**	**N**
I. Pain / nausea adequately controlled			
II. Oxygen therapy discontinued			
III. Patient able to meet hygiene needs with moderate assistance			
IV. Bed / chair rest - walking around bed area only / wheeled to toilet			
V. Tolerating acceptable level of diet and oral fluids			
VI. Anxiety level within acceptable limit			

[4] Transfer to the medical ward will usually occur approx. 24 hours after admission to CCU, and Stage 2 care will therefore usually be carried out while on the medical ward. However if transfer at this time is inappropriate due to the patient's condition please document care on UPR and return to Pathway when Stage 2 care is appropriate. If transfer is delayed for 'staff' or 'system' reasons Stage 2 care which could appropriately be carried out can be signed off while patient is on CCU.

[5] The length of each stage will vary depending on patient's condition. Normally patients will move on to following stage each day, however if this is not appropriate please use UPR to document any further care and return to Pathway when ready to commence next stage.

NAME……………………………………………….. Unit No………………………………

Medical interventions:	Dr's signature
• Review symptom control / vital signs	
• Review medication	
• Exercise ECG arranged for day 6	

Multidisciplinary notes for Stage 2	Sig/designation

STAGE 3	Date commenced Stage 3 care ………………………..		

Nursing interventions:	E	L	N
• BP and HR recorded 4 hourly			
• Refer to dietician if diabetic			
GOALS: *If not met please document in UPR*			
I. Patient able to meet hygiene needs with minimal assistance			
II. Walking one way either to or from the toilet with rest on bed as necessary			
III. Patient pain free			
IV. Anxiety level within acceptable limits			

Medical interventions:	Dr's signature
• Review symptom control / vital signs	
• Review medication	

Multidisciplinary notes for Stage 3	Sig/designation

NAME……………………………………………….. Unit No……………………………….

STAGE 4 Date commenced Stage 4 ……/…../…….			
Nursing interventions:	E	L	
• BP and HR recorded 4 hourly			
GOALS: *If not met please document details in UPR*			
I. Patient able to meet hygiene needs without assistance			
II. Walking both ways to and from the toilet with rest as necessary on bed or chair			
III. Patient pain free			
IV. Anxiety level within acceptable limits			
Medical interventions:	Dr's signature		
• Review symptom control / vital signs			
• Review medication			
• Departmental x-ray booked			
(This is not necessary if previous departmental x-ray already performed - see Section 1c)			
• Sub cut heparin injections continued			
Multidisciplinary notes for Stage 4	Sig/designation		

STAGE 5 Date commenced Stage 5 ……/…../…….			
Nursing interventions:	E	L	
• BP and HR recorded 4 hourly			
GOALS: *If not met please document details in UPR*			
I. Patient able to shower or bath as preferred			
II. Walking freely around ward area			
III. Patient pain free			
IV. Anxiety level within acceptable limits			

NAME.. Unit No.....................................

Medical interventions:	Dr's signature
• Review symptom control / vital signs	
• Review medication	
• TTO's prescribed including Statins if cholesterol level is greater than 6 mmols/litre	
Multidisciplinary notes for Stage 5	Sig/designation

STAGE 6 Date commenced Stage 6 ..../...../.......			
	E	**L**	**N**
• BP and HR recorded 4 hourly			
• Relatives informed of discharge			
• GP informed of discharge			
GOALS: *If not met please document details in UPR*			
I. Patient able to shower or bath as preferred			
II. Walk flight of stairs under supervision or exercise ECG (if appropriate)			
III. Patient pain free			
IV. Anxiety level within acceptable limits			
V. Understanding of information checked by CNS-HD or ward staff if CNS-HD not available			

ECG Technicians Report:	Signature

NAME.. Unit No....................................

Medical intervention:	Dr's signature
• Review symptom control / vital signs	
• Review medication	
• Review 'Exercise Test' results **RESULT**......................................	
• Blood taken for FBC and C&E	
• Pre - discharge 12 lead ECG arranged	
• Ensure "Risk Factors" have been identified in UPR	

Multidisciplinary notes for Stage 6	Sig/designation

DISCHARGE CHECK LIST

Prior to discharge please ensure patient has the following:

TTO's including GTN and compliance card   ❑

Streptokinase Card   ❑

OPD for 6 weeks   ❑

Letter for GP   ❑

Letter for D/N   ❑

Exercise test appointment card (if appropriate)   ❑

Warfarin card / date of next appointment   ❑

Information booklet - Take Heart given to patient   ❑

DATE OF DISCHARGE HOME ..../...../.......

OUTCOMES
On discharge please complete Section B on outcome form at the back of the Pathway

NAME..   Unit No...................................

ALL STAFF COMPLETING PATHWAY MUST COMPLETE THE FOLLOWING

Name (Block Capitals)	Signature	Initials	Designation

Dr A Miller

Amended February 1999

Review February 2000

CHEST PAIN / SUSPECTED / CONFIRMED MYOCARDIAL INFARCTION

OUTCOME FORM   Unit No..................

SECTION A *(To be completed by nursing staff prior to patient leaving CCU)*

There is a wealth of evidence to show that early administration of thrombolytic therapy to patients with acute MI reduces mortality and morbidity.
Collection of the following information will allow us to measure how successfully we are achieving this aim.

Time / date of onset of pain or other major symptoms	
Time / date of call for help (either GP or ambulance)	
Time / date of arrival in A&E department	
Time / date of commencement of thrombolytic therapy	

Was this a "Barn Door" presentation?   Yes ☐   No ☐

i.e. typical history, with ECG evidence of ST evaluation or LBBB thought to be new and no contraindications

Which thrombolytic agent did patient receive?   Streptokinase ☐   Reteplase ☐   None ☐

If none please give brief details

....

Did patient suffer any adverse effects from thrombolysis?   Yes ☐   No ☐

If yes please give brief details

....

SECTION B (*To be completed by Dr on discharge)*

This additional information will be used to measure adherence to guidelines, both local and national.

- Have beta blockers been prescribed as discharge medication?   Yes ☐   No ☐
  If not please give reason
  ....

- Has patient had an exercise test while in hospital?   Yes ☐   No ☐
  If not please give reason
  ....

- How many days has patient spent in hospital? ....
  If longer than 6 days please give reason
  ....

Please detach this page from pathway once completed and send to:
Bev Woodcock
Clinical Audit Facilitator

Appendix 3

Integrated care pathway for day case cardiac catheters

Papworth Hospital NHS Trust

Reviewed 1st January 1999

PAPWORTH HOSPITAL NHS TRUST
INTEGRATED CARE PATHWAY

Day Case Catheters (3)

1

L.O.S 1 day (0 Night)   WARD ....

(Addressograph) NAME HOSPITAL NO.	LIKES TO BE KNOWN AS:
ADDRESS	MARITAL STATUS AGE OCCUPATION
GP DOB	Religion
DATE/ TIME OF ADMISSION CONSULTANT	NEXT OF KIN RELATIONSHIP ADDRESS
DATE OF DISCHARGE	
NAME AND SIGNATURE OF WARD NURSE (please print)	TELEPHONE NUMBER
	TRANSPORT OWN or HOSPITAL
REASON FOR ADMISSION	By Who _____
ALLERGIES (Write "NIL KNOWN" if no allergies)	Time of Collection _____

ABBREVIATIONS ON PATHWAY

appt -	Appointment	(C)	Cardiographer
BP -	Blood Pressure	(CL)	Clerk
CXR -	Chest X-Ray	(CT)	Cardiac Technician
ECG -	Electrocardiograph	(D)	Doctor
L.O.S -	Length of Stay	(N)	Nurse
Pre-Med -	Pre -Operative Medication	(Ph)	Pharmacist
Pt -	Patient	(R)	Radiographer
		(RDA)	*Radiology Department Assistant*
		(S)	Support Worker

This ICP is intended as a guideline only. Each person is an individual and responses may vary.
If you have any questions, talk to a member of the team.

ABROGATION OF HOSPITAL'S LIABILITY

I am aware that personal property including money, not handed to the Hospital for safe keeping is retained at my own risk and that the hospital will accept no responsibility for the loss of, or damage to, personal property of any kind in whatever way the loss or damage may occur, unless deposited for safe custody.

Signed (Patient)   ....

Witness   ....

Date   ....

Form to be signed by patient declining to deposit cash and/or valuables for safekeeping.

Reviewed 1st January 1999

2

PAPWORTH HOSPITAL NHS TRUST
INTEGRATED CARE PATHWAY
Day Case Catheters

Patient Addressograph Label
(minimum of Name & Hospital Number)

Each entry must be Signed, Designation stated, Dated & Timed.

Consultant _____	CCS Classification	NYHA Classification
Unit _____	0 asymptomatic	1 asymptomatic
Admit _____	1 AP on strenuous exertion	2 slight limitation, mild SOB on ordinary activity
Discharge _____	2 slight limitation, AP on ordinary activity	3 marked limitation, SOB on minimal exercise
	3 marked limitation, AP on minimal exertion	4 inability to to carry out any activity, SOB at times at rest
	4 rest pain	

HISTORY (to be completed by Doctor)
        Cardiac History

Risk Factors (to be completed by Doctor/or Nurse)

Smoking _____ (Never/ex<5yrs/Current(amount and yrs)
Diabetes _____ (NIDDM/IDDN)   Blood Sugar (BM) _____
Total Cholesterol _____ mmol/l
_____ date
Hypertension _____ (Y/N), yr diagnosed)
Family History IHD _____ (1^0 rel <60yrs)
Has the patient any broken areas of skin yes / no   if yes start care plan

Exercise _____

Stress _____

Diet _____

MRSA Risk

Patient is an MRSA Carrier Yes/ No
Has been an inpatient on a ward/nursing home with MRSA outbreak Yes/ No
Has been an Inpatient in the Last 3 months Yes/ No
If yes to any of the above START MRSA standard & inform personnel if patient going for tests

Nurse's Signature .... **Date** .... **Time** ....

Reviewed 1st January 1999

3   Each entry must be Signed, Designation stated, Dated & Timed.

OTHER MEDICAL HISTORY

Family History/Social History   *(to be completed by Doctor/or Nurse)*
                Occupation (to include job pre retirement)
                Alcohol (U/wk)

CURRENT MEDICATION   (if patient is on Warfarin please send urgent INR)

ALLERGIES/Sensitivities (+nature of reaction)

EXAMINATION (to be completed by Doctor)
                (Pre-Procedure Observations on page 9 to be carried out by Nurse)
                Alert Operator if BP above 170/100, any pulses absent, BM greater than 15mmol, O_2 sats less than 90%

                requires more than 3 pillows, pain at rest in last month or if INR greater than 1.8

Reviewed 1st January 1999

PAPWORTH HOSPITAL NHS TRUST
INTEGRATED CARE PATHWAY
Day Case Catheters

Patient Addressograph Label
(minimum of Name & Hospital Number)

Each entry must be Signed, Designation stated,Dated & Timed.

INVESTIGATIONS PLANNED

Doctor's advice to patient and explanation + risks of any procedure

Comments / Concerns of patient

Doctor's Signature_____ Designation _____ Date_____ Time _____

INVESTIGATIONS PERFORMED

Doctor's Signature_____ Designation _____ Date_____ Time _____

RESULTS OF INVESTIGATIONS

5   Each entry must be Signed, Designation stated,Dated & Timed.

MANAGEMENT STRATEGY

Treatment to be   Medical   Surgical   Angioplasty
(Please Ring)

                                         Surgeon............................   Priority   1   2   3
                                                                                     (Please Ring)

                                         Referral sent Yes/ NO
                                         Date...............................

Doctor's Signature _____   Designation _____   Date _____ Time _____

Surgical Referral Comments

Doctor's Signature _____   Designation _____   Date _____ Time _____

MEDICATION CHANGE ON DISCHARGE

Doctor's Signature _____   Designation _____   Date _____ Time _____

FOLLOW UP APPOINTMENT

Reviewed 1st January 1999

PAPWORTH HOSPITAL 7

24 hour Prescription Chart

Patient Addressograph Label
(minimum of Name & Hospital Number)

DATE...

WARD...

Drug Allergies/ Sensitivities(or NIL KNOWN)
Dr's Signature...

1. This chart applies only for the 24 hours shown.
2. If the patient requires admission, all treatment must be rewritten on the usual prescription chart.

PRE-MEDICATION AND ONCE ONLY PRESCRIPTIONS

Drug (Approved Name)	Dose	Route	Time to be given	Doctors Signature	Time Given	Signature

REGULAR PRESCRIPTIONS (GIVEN OR TAKEN DURING 24 HOURS ADMISSION)

Drug (Approved Name)	Dose	Route	Frequency (8, 12, 14, 18, 22)	Doctors Signature	Stop OR Continue	Times Given or Taken (Please use initials) 8	12	14	18	22	8

Reviewed 1st January 1999

PAPWORTH HOSPITAL
DAY CASE WARD
INFORMATION ABOUT SELF-ADMINISTRATION OF DRUGS AND
PATIENT ASSESSMENT & CONSENT FORM

8

The admitting nurse with your agreement has decided that whilst you are here you may take your own drugs.
It is not compulsory .

If you agree to take your own medicines you will be asked to sign below together with the nurse who is assessing you and the pharmacist .

HERE ARE A FEW GUIDELINES TO HELP YOU :

1.   Whilst in the Day Case Ward you will have The opportunity to discuss your drug therapy with
             nursing or pharmacy staff - the pharmacist visits the ward daily.

2.   We aim to help you understand the purpose of your drugs, any possible side effects and
             how to take them safely and understand more about your condition and general health / well being.

HOW THE SYSTEM OPERATES :

1.   The Pharmacist who takes your medication history (or a Nurse) will check you have all the
             correct medication with you.

2.   Continue taking your own tablets.

3.   Please keep your medication out of sight of other patients and visitors, locked in your bedside locker.

4.   If you are taking any other medication which has not been written on the prescription overleaf
             please tell the pharmacist or nursing staff. It is important that ALL your medication is charted,
             since the addition of any new medication may interfere with the action of other drugs
                            you are already taking.

5.   If you are prescribed any new medication as a result of your procedure you will be supplied
             with 7 days of medication by the pharmacy and further supplies should be obtained from
                            your GP in the usual way.

6.   Always sign with   *your initial,*   for each dose of your medication taken on this prescription chart.

I have read this information sheet and agree to take my own medicines
whilst on the Day Case Ward.

Signed:_____

Date: _____

I have discussed the self-administration of medicines with the above patient
and assessed their suitability to participate and checked medication.

Nurses Signature:_____

Pharmacist Signature_____

DRUGS TO TAKE HOME   (Maximum 7 days supply)
Please make sure you have indicated on the Drug Chart overleaf which drugs are to continue OR stop.

Drug (Approved Name)	Dose	Route	Frequency	No. of Days	Doctor's Signature	Additional Instructions	Pharmacy

Reviewed 1st January 1999

9

PAPWORTH HOSPITAL
INTEGRATED CARE PATHWAY
Day Case Catheters
L.O.S 1 day (0 Night)

Patient Addressograph Label
(minimum of Name & Hospital Number)

	Pre Procedure Date:					Date: Sig	Date: Sig
	Record Apex, Blood pressure, Height, Weight and BM if patient is Diabetic　(N)						
Pre - Procedure **Observations (N)**	Apex	BP	Height	Weight	BM		
	Diabetic　　　Yes / No　　　if yes Diet　/　Tablet /　Insulin　(N)						
	If pt is a Diabetic on Insulin carry out BM test 2 hourly or if symptomatic whilst Nil by Mouth (N)						
Clinical Assessment	Asthma　　　Yes / No　　(N)						
	Epilepsy　　　Yes / No　　if Yes Last attack　　　　　(N)						
	Bronchitis　　Yes / No　　if yes　O2 Sats＿＿＿＿＿(N)						
	Migraines　　Yes / No　　(N)						
Care & Activity	Check patient has shaved　　(N)						
	Dentures present　　　　　Yes / No　(N)						
	Jewellery　　　removed　/　taped　(please circle)　(N)						
	Remove Makeup　　(N)						
	Patient in a Gown　　(Ask patient if wish to wear Paper Pants)　　(N)						
Medication	Take Morning Drugs　(unless patient is a Diabetic)　(N)						
	Continue Drugs as usual　unless patient is a Diabetic　(N)						
	On Anti-coagulants　Yes / No　Warfarin/ Aspirin　(N)						
	if on Warfarin request URGENT check of　INR (N)						
	Get result RUNG to ward.　　　　　Result............................(N)						
	Premedication needed　　　　Yes / No						
	if YES give at..........................　　(N)						
Safety	Note Allergies on Prescription Chart　　*or write nil known* (D)						
	Ensure informed Consent obtained　　　(D)						
	Check consent signed　(N)						
	Check Name Band is correct　(N)						
	Apply Red allergy Band as necessary (N)						
	Consent for self medication　(N)						
Teaching/ Psychological Support	Explain Procedures　(N)						
	Explain factors affecting Haematoma formation, including						
	Bedrest for 4 hours　(N)						
	NOT to drive for 24hrs post procedure　(N)						
	NO lifting for 2 Days　(N)						
	Assess patients understanding of factors affecting Haematoma formation　(N)						
	Explain Integrated Care Pathway　(N)						
Admission/ Discharge Plan	Book with X-Ray　(CL)						
	Write to patient and send Information Leaflet (CL)						
	Request Notes and X-Rays　(CL)						
	Check transport home is available　(N)						
	Check Relative/ Friend able to stay the night　　(N)						
	JUST PRIOR TO GOING FOR PROCEDURE						
	Check Notes present　(RDA)						
	ECG printout present　(RDA)						
	Check Consent present　(RDA)						
Diet	*Nil by Mouth for 2 hrs pre procedure　(N)*						
Investigations	ECG　(C/N)						
	Bloods　　　　　FBC　U& E's　　LFT's　　X.Match						
	Cholesterol　Glucose						

Doctor ＿＿＿＿＿＿＿　　　　　　　　　　　　　**Please write full signature**

Clinic Nurse ＿＿＿＿＿＿＿　　　　　Ward Nurse ＿＿＿＿＿＿＿

Radiology Department Assistant ＿＿＿＿＿＿＿

Reviewed 1st January 1999

10

Patient Addressograph Label
(minimum of Name & Hospital Number)

PAPWORTH HOSPITAL
INTEGRATED CARE PATHWAY
Day Case Catheters
L.O.S 1 day (0 Night)

	Left Heart Catheter		
			SIG
Clinical Assessment			

Care & Activity	Record Puncture Site (Please Circle side, site & artery or vein)
	Left Right
	                                        Artery Vein
	                                                        Femoral Radial Brachial
	
	Specific Instructions for Post Procedure Care
	Femoral Route
	Apply pressure to site for at least 10 minutes & until Haemostasis has been achieved (D / CT)
	
	Post Radial Catheter Wrist Tourniquet applied at _____
	or
	Post Percutaneous Brachial Catheter Wrist Tourniquet applied at _____
	
	Other Specific Care Required
	--- 	
	--- 	
	--- 	
	--- 	
	--- 			

Medication	Lignocaine 1% Marcaine 0.75% Niopam Contrast media Total Amount in mls........................ (N) Hepsal Flush (N)		
	Diazemuls	Diazemuls	Other
	Heparin	Heparin	
	Intra-Coronary GTN	Intra-Coronary GTN	
	Intra-Coronary GTN	Intra-Coronary GTN	
Safety	Monitor ECG (CT) Time Start.............................. Time Finish................................ Diamentor................................. Screening Time.........................		
Teaching/ Psychological Support	Teach Patient to self monitor puncture site (N)		
Discharge Plan	Return to ward when Haemostasis achieved (D) Taken to ward by Radiology Department Assistant		
Diet	Nil by Mouth		
Investigations	X-Ray Fluoroscopy + acquisition + storage of Radiographic information (R)		

Name in Block Letters	Please write full signature
Doctor	
X-Ray Nurse	
Radiographer	
Cardiac Technician	

Reviewed 1st January 1999

PAPWORTH HOSPITAL
INTEGRATED CARE PATHWAYS

Patient Addressograph Label
(minimum of Name & Hospital Number)

RECORD OF STERILE PACKS USED

Date	WARD
Procedure	

STAFF (All names to be printed and Designation given)	
Operators	Nurses
Signature of Circulating Nurse	Print Name

Please stick labels of all packs used below.

Reviewed 1st January 1999

PAPWORTH HOSPITAL
INTEGRATED CARE PATHWAY
Day Case Catheters
L.O.S 1 day (0 Night)

Patient Addressograph Label
(minimum of Name & Hospital Number)

	Post Left Heart Catheter (Ward)	SIG
Clinical Assessment	1/2hrly BP, Apex, pedal/radial pulse and check wound site for 2hrs (N) Consultant to give patient results (D) Operator to generate summary (D)	

Post Left Heart Catheter Observations *Femoral or Brachial Stab*

Hours post procedure	Apex	BP	Groin/ Site	Pedal /Radial Pulse present
On return				
Pre Sheath Removal				
1/2hr				
1hr				
1& 1/2hrs				
2hrs				

Care & Activity	Sheath removed on Ward YES / NO (N)
	 Time sheath removed .... (N)
	 Apply pressure to site for at least 10 minutes & until Haemostasis has been achieved (N/D/ CT)
	 Lay Flat until sheath removed & then for 1 hr until................................... (N)
	 Bedrest after sheath removal for a total of *2* or 3 or 4 hrs until............................ (N)
	
	 Examine Groin/ Site before **Discharge**, (N)
	 refer to Doctor if :
	         Wound still oozing ++ post procedure
	         Haematoma / Swelling present
	         Lack of adjacent pulse (N)
	
	 Post Radial Angography
	 Remove Arm Tourniquet on return to Ward Time......................................(N)
	 Loosen gradually Wrist Tourniquet 1hour after applied Time...........................(N)
	 Remove completely when haemostasis achieved
	 Patient can mobilise when feels able usually when tourniquet off. (N)

Medication	Patient is Self Medicating, check is continuing drugs as usual (N) Any Change in medication Yes / No if Yes explain change (N) Dispense TTO,s for change of medication if required (N)
Safety	Remind patient to get Medication locked away between taking drugs. (N)
Teaching/ Psychological Support	Teach patient to self monitor puncture site after sheath removal (N) Explain results & future treatment options to patient & family (N) Explain to patients for Valve surgery that must have 6monthly Dental treatment (N) Patients for Heart Surgery must have Body Mass index done.............(N) if BMI over 25 pt told of risk to wound healing & told to lose weight, *GP* informed.(N) Give Discharge advice sheet (N)
Discharge Plan	Nurse to write discharge letter (N) Give copy of *GP* discharge letter to patient (N) Give "Patients Guide to Cardiac Surgery" if for surgery & tell to bring when come to Pre-Admmission Clinic (N) If Brachial Sutures give Suture letter & tell Pt to book appt at GP Surgery on .... (N) Explain to patient will ring in one week. (Record Date on Data Collection form) (N/ S)
Diet	Feed as soon as patient wishes (N)
Investigations	

Please write full signature

AM Nurse	
PM Nurse	
Cardiac Technician	

Day After Procedure:	Date............................
Make Follow up Appointment (S)	
	Signature...

Reviewed 1st January 1999

VARIANCE TRACKING SHEET 12

Patient Addressograph Label
(minimum of Name & Hospital Number)

Day Case Catheters

Date	Time	Variance & Reason for it Could include Extra Drugs given OR Catheters) (Or comments about care unlikely to affect stay)	Variance (Or N/A)	Signature	Action Taken	Signature

Transfer to Ward:

Next of Kin	Aware		Not Aware
Property Checked and Documented	Yes		No
Does Transport need to be arranged	Yes		No

Comment:

Signature :   Designation

Medical		**Drugs**	
B8	Haematoma	C2	Drugs not given
B9	Bleeding post Cardiac Catheter	C6	Premed given late
M11	Angina	C11	Premed given in Department
M13	Bradycardia	C13	Patient is not Self Medicating
M5	Ventricular Tachycardia	**Other**	
F3	Nausea	O6	Extra Investigation
N3	Peripheral nerve injury	O10	Other
N5	Vasal Vagal Attack	**Community**	
Z5	Procedure Cancelled as Pt unwell	A5	Transport Delay
C11	Reaction to Contrast Medium	A6	Transport not Booked
Equipment		A8	OPA not booked
E1	Notes not present	A9	Unable to book OPA
E2	X-Rays not present	A11	Staying in with Medical Problems
E3	No Consent	A11s	Staying in for Surgery
		A11i	Staying in for extra investigations

Staff
S1 Doctor decision
S3 Doctor Late

Index